PLANNING FOR WELLNESS^{sm}
A Guidebook for Achieving Optimal Health
Second Edition

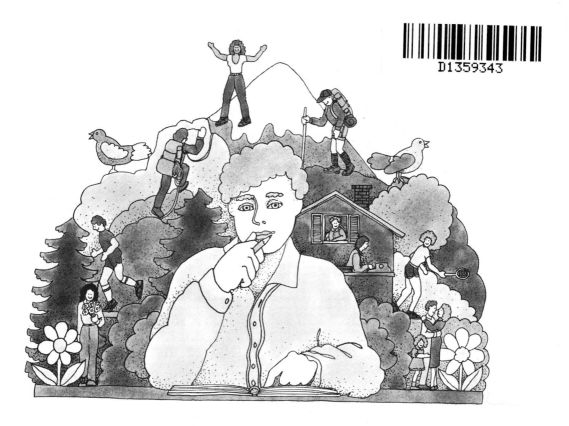

Donald B. Ardell, Ph.D. and Mark J. Tager, M.D.

Illustrated by Nancy Olson

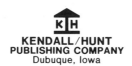

KENDALL/HUNT
PUBLISHING COMPANY
Dubuque, Iowa

Cover photo: Kristen Finnegan

sm 1982 as used throughout this text, *Planning for Wellness,* is a
service mark of Drs. Mark Tager and Donald Ardell. Registration
pending.

B   402717   01

Dedication

To Jack LaLanne and Johnny Kelley—for inspiration.

To Jeanne and Jon, ages 17 and 13, respectively, for showing the effortless side of wellness.

To Jane Fonda—for popularizing wellness and showing how 45-year-old bodies can look given a bit of attention.

To all the hospital administrators, planners, physicians, nurses, and others who are taking risks in order to pioneer creative pathways to wellness programming.

To Frederick Anlyan, M.D., Steve Willard, Douglas Strain, Gary Boyles, Ph.D., and Marvin Goldberg, M.D., who have provided guidance over the years.

And, last but not least, to Sam Scherzer, age five, whose displeasure at having to go to kindergarten for the first time was quoted by Herb Cain in the *San Francisco Chronicle*. "Golly," Sam pouted, "I can tie my shoes, stand on my head, snap my fingers, and ride a two-wheeler—what else is there to learn?"

Contents

Preface

This book is a simple, workable, and—we hope—enjoyable approach to personal wellness planning. When you finish it, you will be ready to write and carry out your own lifestyle plan for optimal health and improved personal performance.

Planning for Wellness begins by summarizing the wellness concept and showing how it differs both from the traditional medical model and from alternative health care approaches. Next, we define the steps involved in personal wellness planning. We will encourage you to select a health improvement goal and will guide you toward reaching it. In the Skills section we have provided the information on fitness, stress management, and nutrition necessary to carrying out your plan. Finally, with the aid of some challenging exercises, you will examine how to develop the supportive environments at home, work, and play that will help you maintain your personal wellness goal.

There is more to **Planning for Wellness,** however, than just getting yourself healthy. Wellness really begins to happen when individuals come together as a community and work toward a shared purpose with confidence and optimism. This group interaction fosters a climate which can make your efforts to become well more meaningful and more successful. The community's purposes transcend individual gratification, setting in place deep-seated social and even spiritual missions. The goals of the community then become the highest, strongest, and most enduring reasons for keeping on a path to personal wellness.

As you work through this guidebook, we will be encouraging you to join with others to form systems of mutual support. We will suggest strategies to enlist the aid of your friends, family members, and co-workers.

Welcome to **Planning for Wellness.**

Chapter

1

The Wellness Concept

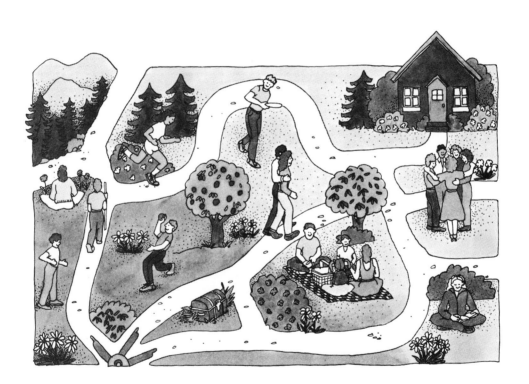

Wellness—What Is It?

Wellness is many things. It is, first of all, *a very special kind of lifestyle*. It is a lifestyle you shape for yourself—consciously—to reach your best possibilities for well-being. It entails a focus on the joys of living life to the fullest.

One purpose of a wellness lifestyle is to ascend to whatever heights are within your sights. Another is to increase your capacity to perceive and seek out new heights. To do so requires an understanding of how wellness differs from other approaches to health.

Prevention strategies (such as stop-smoking programs, or alcohol and drug abuse programs) have, as the terms suggests, focused on avoiding illness. The same is true of health education, prospective medicine, preventive health care, and similar established efforts. They are fine as far as they go, but their orientation is different from the wellness concept; the latter begins where the others leave off.

You may be a smoker. You may drink more alcohol than you know is good for you. You may be concerned about your weight. There may be other "problem" areas that you would like to address with a wellness plan. Wellness can resolve these problems for you. But a wellness lifestyle can do much more for you than just help you stop smoking, drink less, or become slim. A wellness lifestyle can help you achieve positive states of vitality far beyond what you thought possible.

Another term which some people confuse with wellness is "holistic health." Are these concepts the same? Not by a long shot.

Technically, holism is a philosophical approach that can be applied to almost any field. It implies an effort to grasp the "big picture," to look at the way various parts come together to create a new "whole." The term has been applied to astronomy, biology, education, business, and even military operations. But it is not the concept of holism we wish to distinguish from wellness, it is its current application to health.

Holistic health is treatment-oriented. As it is usually presented, it involves non-surgical, non-drug methods for healing. Herbal remedies, touch therapies, colonic irrigations, chiropractic and naturopathic programs are illustrative of the range of treatments falling under this banner. Practitioners of holistic health remedies are sometimes physicians, but more often are not. Either way, holistic health programs rely upon a practitioner for diagnosis and treatment.

In contrast, wellness does not require a practitioner to make it happen; it is not a treatment program relying on outside agents. It is a lifestyle which only **you** can make happen.

Wellness is also a *social movement, with powerful economic implications.*
The movement has consequences for schools, churches, families, and worksites.
It may expand to affect all areas of society. As a movement, wellness holds
potential for cutting health care costs through advances in the public's health
status, appropriate use of the medical care system, and the development of
strong social systems that reinforce personal responsibility for health.

Although wellness is a relatively new development, it has its own history,
dating back to the efforts of Halbert L. Dunn, M.D., in the late 1950s. Dunn
was a distinguished administrator, physician, lecturer, and writer. He won many
awards and honors in his field of epidemiology and public health. However, it
was in his retirement years that he made his contribution to the wellness movement that was to begin in the mid-seventies, after his death at age 80. In his
little-acclaimed but highly influential collection of lectures entitled *High Level
Wellness,* published in 1960, Dunn addressed himself to the interrelationship
of all living things, the value of lifestyle, and the importance of viewing and
promoting health as an elevated state of superb functioning. The book inspired
a young medical intern a decade after its publication and motivated him to
establish a "wellness center" where people could be encouraged to pursue health
apart from illness treatment. That intern became the nation's first wellness
physician. His name was John Travis. The work of Dr. Travis, the publication
of *High Level Wellness: An Alternative to Doctors, Drugs, and Disease* (Ardell, Rodale Press, 1977), and the adoption of the term by such influential figures as Dr. William Hettler of the University of Wisconsin, Stevens Point, and
Dr. Robert Allen of the Human Resources Institute, among others, led to the
rapid spread of the term "wellness."

The next breakthrough was the establishment of the first wellness program
by a major medical center, Swedish Hospital of Denver, Colorado. Less than
a year after the opening and successful marketing of the Swedish Wellness
Center, other progressive institutions followed the hospital's lead. In just a two-
year span, hundreds of innovative groups organized their own forms of wellness
programming. Among the results of these efforts were the Center for Health
Promotion of the American Hospital Association, the Frost Valley YMCA
wellness summer camp programs, the Wallingford Wellness Project for Senior
Citizens, several corporate wellness institutes, the Newark Urban Council for
Inner City Youth, and university-based centers and conferences.*

Wellness is a *value issue*—a reflection of the inner person, one aspect of the
search for meaning and purpose in life's activities. Thus you will find as much
emphasis in this guidebook on psychological advances as on ways to fashion

---

*For a fuller discussion of 23 such centers, see *14 Days to a Wellness Lifestyle,* Mill Valley: Whatever Press,
1982.

great bodies. In addition to a personal wellness plan, at the end of your encounter with *Planning for Wellness* you will have a profile of what it means to be a truly healthy person.

But we also like to think of this encounter as a game—a game with rules (or at least guidelines), players, spectators, and ways to measure progress. The idea of this game is to help the participants experience a full measure of zest for living, and to think of themselves as deserving nothing less than a wellness lifestyle.

So let's get on with the game. Here are some additional guidelines which we'll acquaint you with as we go.

- A view of health as more than non-illness
- A reassessment of an earlier decision
- A five-dimensional program
- An emphasis on individuality
- An orientation toward experiential learning
- A different way of using the "health" care system
- A conscious commitment to excellence
- Changing expectations
- A focus on personal wellness planning

Health Is a Great Deal More Than Non-Sickness

Surveys have shown that people think of themselves as healthy if they are not in pain, are not suffering from a cold or the flu, and are not otherwise impaired in any way that impedes their "normal" functioning. At times the medical system promotes this view: if no illness conditions are found in the traditional check-up or annual physical exam, the patient gets a "clean bill of health."

This point of view is hazardous to your health! There is more to health than not being sick. In the final analysis, you are the one who will have to decide what constitutes "health" for you—in what specific ways, health goes beyond the absence of illness/disease.

As you go through *Planning For Wellness,* we would like you to put aside any thoughts about heart disease, cancer, high blood pressure, or warts, and focus instead on the positive motivators which for you make life a joy.

This commitment to the positive is at the heart of a wellness lifestyle. In the pages that follow, you will find very little about the hazards of "worseness" lifestyles, because we do not believe scare tactics can sustain your initial motivation to change.

Of course, there are some fundamentals concerning health risks which you should recognize. No doubt you already do. However, just in case you have not been keeping up with medical journals, health books, diet magazines, or daily newspapers, here are some health hazard statistics:

- Of the ten leading causes of death in the U.S., at least seven could be substantially reduced if people improved just five aspects of their lifestyle: diet, smoking, exercise, alcohol, and blood pressure control.
- Smoking cigarettes nearly doubles the risk of heart attack for men.
- Alcohol is a major factor in more than 10% of all deaths in the United States.
- Up to 20% of total cancer mortality may be associated with occupational hazards.
- In 1977, highway accidents killed 49,000 people and led to 1,800,000 disabling injuries. It's estimated that wearing seatbelts can reduce the likelihood of serious injury or death by almost half.
- One in four American girls have had at least one pregnancy by age 19. Approximately 300,000 of these adolescents are under 15.
- Elevated blood pressure affects one in six Americans and contributes to the 500,000 strokes and 1,250,000 heart attacks which occur annually.
- Suicide is the third leading cause of death among teenagers and young adults.

We didn't invent these statistics (if we had, we would have been much more imaginative). They are from *Healthy People: The Surgeon General's Report on Health Promotion and Disease Prevention.* In signing this document, the President of the United States said, "Our fascination with the more glamorous 'pound of cure' has tended to dazzle us into ignoring the often more effective 'ounce of prevention.' "

Our Canadian friends can obtain comparable data from *A New Perspective on the Health of Canadians,* issued by the Ministry of Health and Welfare in 1974.

You might want to go a bit further by completing an informative survey known as a "health risk assessment." A number of groups distribute a low-cost computerized questionnaire filled with similar data on the risks of certain behavior. By completing such a survey, you learn how long you are likely to survive given your current behavior, and what you could gain from reforming your lifestyle in certain ways.

Our focus will be to help you learn more about the dimensions of wellness. The more satisfaction wellness brings you, the stronger will be your commitment to it, and—as the movement spreads—the more plentiful will be the numbers of persons living a "wellness" lifestyle.

A Reassessment of an Earlier Decision

How many times have you heard of a situation like the following: Horatio Hardriver—a sedentary, middle-aged, high-pressure executive—suffers a coronary at a massage parlor. In a tense scene, Horatio is saved thanks to the efforts of three of the masseuses who had taken CPR training and were "on duty" when Horatio had his climactic arrest. After a hectic rush to the hospital, emergency treatment, and months of care and rehabilitation, and $30,000 in hospital and doctor bills, Horatio sees the light. He resolves to change his life-style.

Horatio becomes a swimmer, biker, and proponent of natural foods. He not only stops smoking; he organizes a "non-smoker's rights" group. In addition, he learns to manage stress, becomes a deacon in his church, and leads a successful campaign to close the local massage parlors. In an interview, Horatio declaims, "Having a heart attack may have been the best thing that ever happened to me."

There are a number of terms to describe Horatio's sudden change of heart. Some would call it serendipity; others, familiar with the medical care system, would label it a "teachable moment."

One kind of teachable moment occurs when a person is willing to hear and then act upon messages his or her body may be sending. Other teachable moments can take the form of life crises (e.g., economic reversals, natural calamities) and even positive events (e.g., a new job, new romance, or an unexpected honor).

We are frequently exposed to changes which create potential teachable moments. The secret, of course, is to be alert to such changes, to become listeners, and to adjust to the new situation. The goal of the wellness game is not just to live longer but to lead a life of higher performance. Paying attention to teachable moments is an important part of the game.

Common Physical Teachable Moments

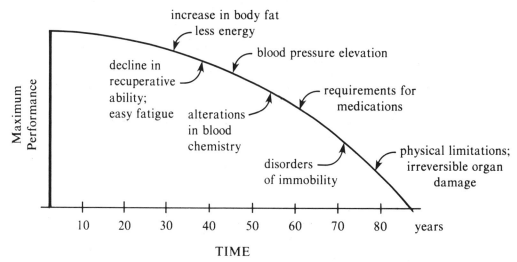

The goal of the wellness game is to shift this curve up and to the right.

We believe many adults made a decision at some point in their lives that achieving and maintaining optimal health was too much trouble. They decided they did not have the time, energy, or ability to pull it off. We also think such decisions were not consciously arrived at, but made by default, in the absence of reinforcement for wellness.

This book has been structured so you can become aware of whether, at some earlier point in life, you made this kind of decision. If you did, you may want to make another kind of decision now—a conscious choice this time to go for nothing less than the best you can be.

We believe that once you know the facts and understand the alternatives, there isn't any contest. If you ever made a decision that optimal functioning was beyond your reach, you have come to the right place—or book.

A Five-Dimensional Program

As with any other specialty, wellness planning has its own tools for change to a healthy lifestyle. A systematic manner for envisioning these tools is the five-dimensional framework shown in the following diagram. These dimensions constitute the five major aspects of a wellness lifestyle.

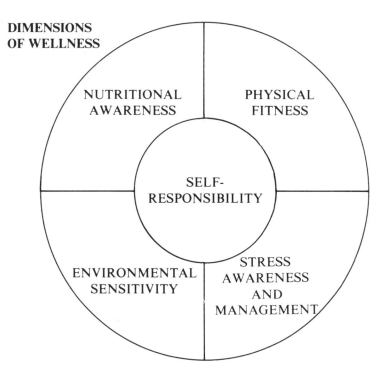

DIMENSIONS OF WELLNESS

NUTRITIONAL AWARENESS

PHYSICAL FITNESS

SELF-RESPONSIBILITY

ENVIRONMENTAL SENSITIVITY

STRESS AWARENESS AND MANAGEMENT

One of these dimensions is more equal than the others. That, of course, is self-responsibility, and for this reason it is placed in the "hub" position on the diagram.

Taking an exaggerated position on the issue, "Who's responsible?" gives you an advantage in the wellness game. For the more you believe yourself to be responsible for what goes well *or* poorly, the more likely you are to act in such a way as to bring about the outcomes you desire. Here are five beliefs which imply a high level of self-responsibility.

- I am in control of my health; doctors, drugs, and medical procedures can only deal with illness states.
- Whether sick or well, I am responsible for my state.
- The main things which affect my health are my attitudes, beliefs, and behaviors.
- If I take care of myself, I can drastically reduce the prospects of illness while dramatically improving my chances of optimal functioning.
- If I lead a wellness lifestyle, I can come close to my best potential and derive great satisfaction from doing so.

If these attitudes are consistent with your current attitudes, you are starting from a position of advantage. If not, do not despair—or go away. By the time you complete *Planning For Wellness* and your own personal wellness plan, you will perceive the benefits of viewing things from such a perspective.

When you come from a position of "I am responsible," you do not waste much time on blaming, making excuses, giving up, or otherwise justifying anything less than your best effort on matters of consequence. As you read *Planning For Wellness,* you might want to keep in mind another question concerning this "hub" dimension of wellness: "What attitude or belief will serve me best in living a wellness lifestyle?" With this query in mind, the benefits of taking responsibility for oneself become more obvious.

Given the pre-eminence of self-responsibility, it must be acknowledged that the other four dimensions *are* essential. In fact, the more you take responsibility for yourself, the deeper your allegiance to the other four dimensions. We'll be discussing these four dimensions in successive chapters.

An Emphasis on Individuality

There is no way we or anyone else can tell you how to live your wellness lifestyle. There are no gurus in the wellness movement, no authority figures who could describe exactly what you ought to do in each of the five dimensions to ensure the highest returns and greatest satisfaction. Books, seminars, and counselors can provide advice, information, and alternatives, but only you can define what wellness is for you. You are unique; there never has and never will again be anyone with your special talents, background, values, and needs—and we respect and celebrate that fact, as did the (anonymous) author of the following verse:

"I am convinced that when I meet my maker, the query will not be: 'Why were you not more like this one or that one?'
No, the Divine Question will be:
Why did you not dream, listen, and love more?
Why did you not create, give, and inspire more?
Why did you not use every precious moment I gave you?
Why were you not more like the great strong person I envisioned when you were conceived?
For I only made one of you."

An Orientation Toward Experiential Learning

This book is set up for your *participation* in wellness planning. Reading about something is one thing; living it is quite another. While both are necessary, only your active involvement can promote your chances for genuine comprehension and commitment. Experiential learning seeks to integrate thoughts, feelings and values with actions. An excellent example of this integration can be seen in the following anecdote:

Mohatma Gandhi, the renowned pacifist, once lectured to the British government on behalf of Indian sovereignty for a solid three hours. During this time he not only kept his audience spellbound, he also did not make a single flaw in his eloquent presentation. At the conclusion of his lecture, his press secretary was beseiged by members of the British press corps, who wanted to know how Gandhi could lecture so flawlessly without a notecard or any other speaking aids.

"It's simple," replied his secretary. "What Gandhi thinks, says, and does are one. You British think one thing, say a second, and do a third. That's why you need notecards to keep track."

Wellness planning seeks to bring your actions into closer harmony with your underlying health values. To do so requires the understanding that comes from experience. Our exercises offer you the chance to learn experientially, by participating in a process of wellness planning.

These exercises are designed for two kinds of experiential learning. One is to record, for your own use, your responses to our questions or invitations. These lists, free associations, rank order choices, and the like, can be written in the book, on a separate notepad, or in your personal journal.

A second option is to share your written account with others. The most valuable phase of any wellness workshop occurs when participants identify in specific ways how the issues connect to their own experience. Each participant comes to realize that others face some of the same dilemmas. This experience leads to group support, creative brainstorming, and new insights. Sharing your responses increases the prospects for your experiential learning.

Therefore, we suggest you try to use the exercises in this book in both ways. Complete every exercise, being sure to write down your responses as well as your reflections on the exercise.

Try not to save time by skipping this activity. Writing your thoughts, feelings, and awarenesses on paper brings to conscious attention the fact you take what you are doing seriously. It forces you to give yourself the attention you richly deserve. Jotting down a response quickly becomes a habit; you become more able to tap the information stored in your subconscious mind.

Then, find a group of persons who will do the same on selected exercises, and share your responses. In this way, you will get more return for yourself and contribute to others in the bargain. You may even find yourself becoming more Gandhi-like, with harmony of thoughts, words, and deeds.

Another Way of Using the "Health" Care System

You can do more for your own health than any physician, hospital, drug, or new medical test can do. Yet you also need to know what modern medicine can do for you.

The figure below illustrates the differences in goals between a wellness program and our health care system.

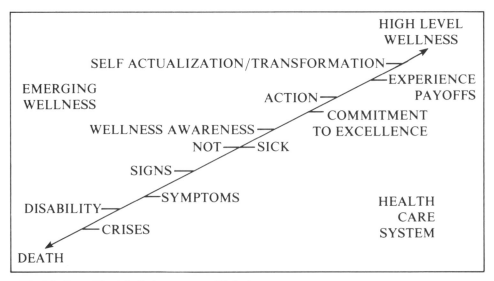

Health *Care*/Health *Enhancement* Dichotomy

The efforts of our medical care system are usually concentrated below the midpoint of the graph. The billions spent on health care each year are targeted toward returning those with signs and symptoms of disease to states of "normal" functioning (i.e., mediocrity).* But the area above the middle line of nonsickness is overlooked. You have a different health goal. Your goal is to move beyond simply "not being sick" toward higher levels of health.

Still, there will be times when even the most faithful wellness advocate becomes ill. (Contrary to popular beliefs, wellness doesn't prevent the common cold, even though it does endow the "patient" with a cheerier attitude.) There will be times when you will need to interact with doctors, hospitals, and pharmacies.

In recent years a wellness movement that emphasizes responsibility for oneself has suggested some guidelines for dealing with the medical system. The movement is titled "medical self-care," and through the efforts of such proponents as Drs. Tom Ferguson (**Medical Self-Care Magazine**), Vickery and Fries *(Take Care of Yourself)*, Keith Sehnert *(How To Be Your Own Doctor Sometimes)*, Don Kemper *(Healthwise Handbook)*, and Joe Graedon *(The People's Pharmacy)*, a series of guidelines have been developed to help you become a "better doctor—sometimes." These guidelines include:

- viewing the physician as an equal partner in the healing process;
- learning to diagnose and treat simple conditions (sprains, sore throats, upset stomachs) at home;
- knowing when a condition requires a specialist's care, and when it can be treated at home;
- getting the most from a doctor's visit by being prepared, assertive, and objective;
- saving money on medications and treatment;
- using over-the-counter medications properly.

The health or medical system should be set up to work in both directions. In addition to learning about self-care, prevention, and wellness, we must learn to make the best use of the system. Modern medicine is a wonderful thing, but there are two problems with how we view it: people expect too much of it, and too little of themselves.

Planning For Wellness will help you make the best of both worlds.

---

*George Sheehan, M.D., author and athlete in his sixties, claims that true normalcy is being the best you can be at any age. Unhappily, most have settled for "accelerated aging" and an attendant "precipitious decline in performance." This, says Sheehan, has given aging a bad name. Most "normals" do not age—they rust. See Dr. George Sheehan, "Medical Advice," *Runner's World,* April 1982, p. 105.

We are, quite frankly, disturbed at some attitudes toward the practice of medicine. Specifically, a story out of Pontiac, Michigan, reported by United Press International (**San Francisco Chronicle,** 2/25/82, p. 28) has us concerned that perhaps things are getting out of hand. It seems that someone in Pontiac (name withheld) was arrested for treating a sick woman "by biting the neck of a freshly killed rooster and sprinkling its blood on the patient's body." As a result, the health practitioner, a "minister" of an unidentified religion working without benefit of accredited health training, has been arrested for "practicing medicine without a license."

License or not, something's wrong here. The person who should be arrested (for gullibility) is the turkey who thought this approach would cure her headaches.

Do you have any bizarre expectations of medical practitioners?

A Conscious Commitment to Excellence

In a story about the devil's treachery (**The Screwtape Letters**),* C. S. Lewis describes Lucifer's efforts to train a protégé to lure souls into Hades. The devil emphasizes throughout the tale that it is not the great failures/calamities/ tragedies that bring men and women to ruin, but little temptations laid out along the way. In a concluding comment in this famous tongue-in-cheek tale, the devil summarizes with these words: "The surest and safest road to hell is the gradual one, soft underfoot, without sudden turnings, without signposts, without milestones."

So it is with our less-than-optimal lifestyles. You can inadvertently end up living a lifestyle of "middle-level mediocrity" or "low-level worseness" without really thinking about it.

Not so with wellness. This kind of pattern comes about and is sustained only through conscious choice, never by accident. In a wellness program, the decision to go for the best within you is always a deliberate choice.

It is important that you not confuse the notion of a commitment to excellence with rigid rules or self denial. Your expectations, hopes and dreams are the fuels which will drive you toward improvement; they can be sources of pain and misery when the expectations themselves are unrealistic.

The conscious commitment to excellence which we are advocating must be tempered with self-acceptance. There is genuine pleasure to be obtained by

*Lewis, **The Screwtape Letters** (New York: Macmillan Co., 1943).

striving to meet high standards. On the other hand, when you strain compulsively, when the goal is unrealistic, when the actual pursuit is mirthless—then the drive to excel becomes self-defeating.

Changing Expectations

Ever heard of Antti Loikkanen? Here is a hint: Antti is a runner who lives in Finland. Now do you have it? Probably not, unless you are related to Mr. Loikkanen—he's not exactly a household word.

What about Roger Bannister? Everybody's heard of the good Dr. Bannister who, in 1954, shattered the four-minute mile barrier for the first time. Until the break-through performance, runners and the interested public believed it could not be done—and therefore it wasn't. Once Bannister demonstrated otherwise, the floodgates were opened. Thousands of sub-four-minute miles have been recorded in the past decade, and the world mark has fallen to the mid three-forties. One runner, John Walker of New Zealand, has himself run more than 70 sub-four-minute miles! In a recent international meet, a runner clocked a time of 3:58.96 (which would have placed him about ten yards ahead of Roger Bannister when he broke the barrier in 1954!) . . . and finished 13th in the race. By now, you probably have figured out his name: Antti Loikkanen.

Wellness is to the usual standard of health what Roger Bannister's run in 1954 was to the four-minute mile: a breakthrough standard.

There are comparable advances to be made in overcoming self-imposed barriers and limitations in daily life. For example:

- The boss comes into your office and declares: "We've got a big problem." What sort of expectation comes to mind? You are waiting for calamitous news. But you could view the "problem" as an opportunity. Why not turn your expectations around?
- You think you are too old to exercise, to change your food habits, and to try relaxation techniques. Besides, even if you did have the time, it probably wouldn't work for you anyway. In this case, once again, the real problem is your expectation.
- Everyone in class says Dr. Flunkum is a brutal grader and her tests are medieval. You have stayed up studying and worrying. But you blow the test. Was your performance affected by your beliefs?

What you expect affects what you get. Wellness encourages you to extend your perspectives—and your reach. If you behave in a way that anticipates health outcomes beyond simply not being sick, your chances for moving beyond the "absence of illness" stage of health are infinitely improved.

By your example, you can infect others with new expectations, too. Before long we could have a veritable epidemic of virulent wellness!

We cannot forget the lesson of the 134-year-old man of the Vilcambamba group in the mountains of Ecuador. After a hard day of farming potatoes on a steep hillside (which greatly fatigued his young interviewer), this spry centurion noted that his stamina was a bit off. In fact, he said, rather wistfully: "Oh, to be 108 again."

A Focus on Personal Wellness

It is not enough to read about good ideas, interesting approaches, and promising alternatives. Eventually you have to make some decisions. These decisions should grow out of a personal assessment of your own expectations and desires. A personal wellness plan is an indispensable step in getting started. It will help you evaluate your purposes, goals, objectives, expected payoffs, and barriers to wellness. We believe you will find the process to be energizing and invaluable. Now that you are an expert on the wellness concept, the time has come to train our attention on the planning process.

Chapter

2

To Be or Not to Be
A Personal Wellness Planner

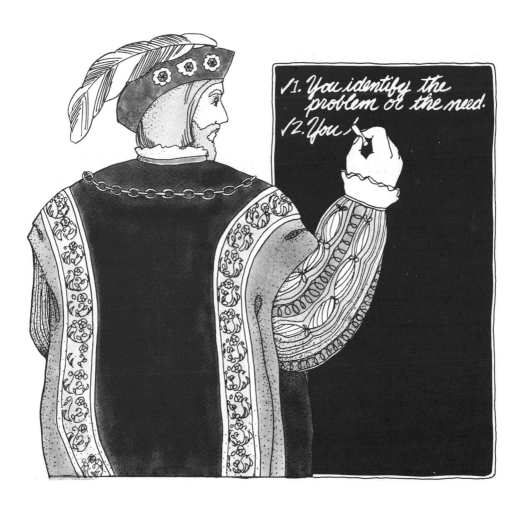

Introduction

For better or worse, you *are* a planner! You may not have given this matter a lot of attention, but you have been engaged in planning for years.

Whether it's shopping, budgeting, transporting the children around town, or getting ready for work each morning, you undoubtedly spend countless hours preparing for your life's many events.

Chances are you don't earn your living by planning. Nevertheless, you in fact do go through the same process that professional planners, regional planners, resource planners, and all other planners follow in detail with the aid of their computers, maps, mountains of data, and political procedures. Here's how the classic planning process works:

1. You identify the problem or need.
2. You brainstorm ideal solutions and desired states.
3. You think about the resources available.
4. You make a choice.
5. You create a plan.
6. You carry out the plan and develop support for maintaining it.
7. You pay attention to how things are going and adjust as necessary.

We are all familiar with this planning process. But when it comes to health, many of us are very poor planners. The result is that Americans, as a people, are less healthy than they could be.

The reasons for this are not really complex. The information we need is not always available, and what information we do have is sometimes disheartening. Moreover, the values we have been taught generally do not support wellness. We are encouraged to pop pills, potions, and powders at the first sign of an ache or feeling of illness. In fact, we pay far more attention to illness than we do to wellness. Yet planning for wellness can be easy and a lot more fun than focusing on the dismal symptoms of constipation, insomnia, headache, and muscle tension.

You do not need to make things complex to get effective results from your planning. Certainly you do not have to spend a fortune on the computers or other technological hardware of the professional planners. But you do need to plan consciously if you want to get the best results. In the quest for wellness, conscious planning versus unaware planning makes all the difference. PLANNING FOR WELLNESS is designed to encourage you to plan more consciously.

Identifying the Problem or Need

1. To prepare you for this step, let's take a closer look at the classic planning process from the standpoint of shaping a wellness lifestyle. Let's start with the idea of *identifying the problem or need*. This is the first step in planning, whether you are doing so as a professional or, as in the present situation, for personal wellness purposes.

A first obstacle for many of us is realizing that we might have a health problem even if we are not sick. Health is not an all-or-nothing, black-vs.-white phenomenon. Our level of wellbeing is constantly in flux, changing from morning to night, from day to day, from year to year.

Are you healthier today than you were last year at this time? About the same? A year from today will your thoughts, feelings, and actions lead you to higher levels of vitality, enjoyment, and effectiveness?

Few people give a thought to their health until something goes wrong, until they become ill. From the viewpoint of wellness, health is much more: if you don't have an abundance of energy and vitality, ample nurturing and constructive relationships, an integrated lifestyle with effective skills to handle life's tensions, a confident sense of purpose and value in life, and if you're not having a great deal of fun— then at least consider that you might have a health problem!

On the following chart we have listed some of the characteristics of wellness and of its unpleasant alternative. Carefully examine these traits. You might want to add some of your own in the spaces provided.

WORSENESS		WELLNESS
−10	**0**	**+10**
low self-esteem	**"normal" health**	positive self-concept
monitor illness signs	absence of illness	monitor wellness signs
focus on disease	no pain	focus on vitality
boredom	not sick	aliveness
fatigue		energy
hostility and blame		calm and accountability
dependency		interdependence
health risk habits		health enhancing behavior
at effect		at cause
no fun		joy
_____		_____
_____		_____

The Wellness/Worseness Continuum

As a means of developing your ability to reach more satisfying states with modest effort, we would like you to complete the following exercise. It will help you decide where you think you are at the start of your *Planning for Wellness* program. It is very important to get a fix on your imagined position before going much further.

The Wellness/Worseness continuum exercise asks you to locate yourself on the scale, and then to respond to a few searching questions we put to you. You should write your answers in the space provided. (If you do not want someone to discover what you have written, respond in some secret code or use a separate sheet of paper.)

Your goal in doing this exercise is to make an honest judgment of how well you *think* you are doing. By thoughtfully addressing a few key questions, you should have a self-inventory that will be useful as an assessment and planning tool.

The first step is quite simple. Place an "X" somewhere on the following line. The line represents a scale of lifestyle behavior ranging from "terrible" on the far left (worseness) to "terrific" on the far right. Consider for a few minutes the qualities by which we have characterized the wellness lifestyle, and then reflect for just a moment on the extent and quality of your attitudes and habit patterns in each of the five basic wellness dimensions. But, don't dwell on the matter. Take 30 seconds, at most.

Is thirty seconds up? Place your X.

−10 −9 −8 −7 −6 −5 −4 −3 −2 −1 0 +1 +2 +3 +4 +5 +6 +7 +8 +9 +10

Here are a few questions to think about. Please write out the first responses that occur to you.

Why did you not make your mark a few places more to the right of the scale?

_____

_____

_____

_____

_____

Have there been times in your life when you would have marked yourself further to the right? If so, how have things changed? Why are you less healthy in your lifestyle habits today?

_____

_____

_____

_____

_____

What are the barriers and obstacles holding you back? Make a list of at least ten, if you can. Take just two minutes. Don't censor yourself—list whatever comes to mind.

_____

_____

_____

_____

Let's take a closer look at the obstacles you have identified. Determine which ones are (1) habits and behaviors, which are (2) thoughts, feelings, and attitudes, and which are (3) existing physical limitations. Now comes the hard part. After categorizing these problems, you need to determine your priorities. How do you decide which obstacles to address first?

Often—especially if your list is long—the process of identifying obstacles or problems can reinforce feelings of hopelessness and negative self-worth. It is easy for the average person to feel overwhelmed, as if he or she needed to change everything at once—stop smoking, drinking, and eating junk food; start exercising and managing stress; improve his or her attitude, job and family situations; _and_ invent another eight hours in the day. Furthermore, all of these changes "must" take place overnight. But changes, especially changes in long-established habits, just do not work that way.

Whichever obstacle you choose to work on, chances are that it will take some time to change. In this connection, there is one additional principle you need to know about wellness:

It doesn't matter what you choose to work on—the key is to be successful.

Wellness is a series of little steps. Every once and awhile it may be possible to make a giant leap. But for the most part, making changes is a process of gradually acquiring confidence, skills, and success over time.

Naturally, you alone can assess the power of each obstacle, the value of each process, and the merit of each course of action. When pondering what to do first, consider the following measures; determine the effects of overcoming each barrier; then, based on how you like to do things, rank those effects:

- Promise of quick success   _____
- Level of energy/initiative needed   _____
- Amount of fun you will have doing it   _____

My Barriers
1. smoking
2. not enough exercise
3. too much responsibility at work
4. long hours on job
5. not enough freedom in work
6. poor diet
7. need to cut loose and have more fun
8. worry about things
9. not enough time

JEAN LEBACK
PORTLAND, OREGON

- Extent that money is needed to get started   _____
- Impact that it will have on your health   _____
- Extent to which the endeavors will enhance your
  self concept   _____
- Time required   _____
- Other (please complete)   _____
-   _____
-   _____

You may find, after considering these measures, that more is involved than logic and pay-off. For example, suppose you listed smoking as a barrier. You are aware that stopping smoking will have the greatest impact on your health, will require a minimum of time, and will enhance your self-concept greatly.

However, you realize that if you go cold turkey, you will have nothing to replace the negative habit. Beginning a jogging program, on the other hand, will also have a major impact on your health, self-concept, and energy level. While it may take a bit more time, you determine that you are *more likely to succeed* at a modest exercise program. Furthermore, success in developing a "positive addiction" to exercise will make it much easier to let go of the cigarette habit in the days, weeks or months to come.

At this point you've probably noticed that you're an expert at listing barriers. Most of us are. In describing what you would like to accomplish, it's essential to consider the up-side probabilities as well. In other words, you now need to brainstorm what **could** be.

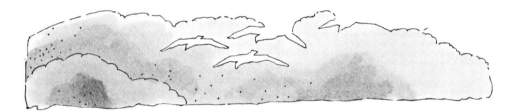

Brainstorming Solutions
and Desired States

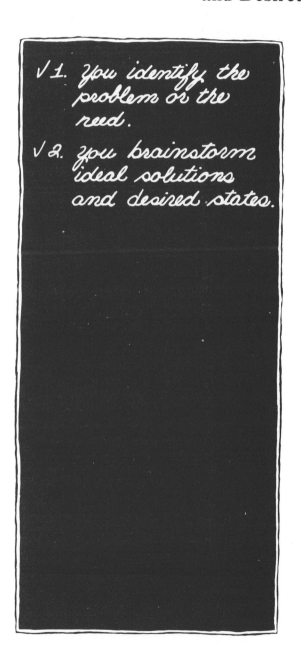

√ 1. You identify the problem or the need.

√ 2. You brainstorm ideal solutions and desired states.

2. Step two in the planning process is to open the floodgates of creative possibilities. This activity requires uninhibited listing of seemingly bizarre, impractical, outlandish, politically untenable, or otherwise too expensive/impossible/utopian fantasy alternatives! The activity is called brainstorming because it involves a torrent of thoughts in a downpour of free-flowing suggestions for a perfect future state.

A striking thing usually happens when individuals and groups engage in brainstorming. Freed from the usual constraints, their imaginations soar. Stranger still, the resulting flow is usually insightful and eventually usable, by no means far-out and ridiculous.

Toward Utopia

What would you be like if you had unlimited time, financial resources, and physical and mental attributes (e.g. virtue in abundance) to create the ultimate you? Specifically:

What could you achieve that you value? (Be ambitious.)

_____

_____

_____

_____

How might you appear, under the best of circumstances?

_____

_____

_____

_____

What would your ideal environment at home and work look like?

_____

_____

_____

What would be your major leisure activities?

_____

_____

_____

_____

What payoffs would you gain from truly concentrating on making wellness a priority in your life? Say that you really worked at developing and carrying out a personal wellness plan for an hour a day for the next six months. What difference would it make? How would you be better off? Be specific. Take five minutes.

_____

_____

_____

_____

_____

Let's assume the fantasies you listed above actually did come about, and they had all the wonderful consequences you imagined. On the continuum listed on the following page place a circle "O" where you think you would be, given total success.

Make one final mark on the continuum. Place one star "*" where you *will* be in two months, two stars "**" in six months, and three stars "***" in one year.

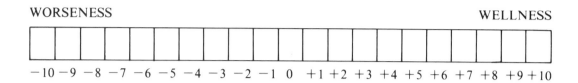

WORSENESS   WELLNESS

-10 -9 -8 -7 -6 -5 -4 -3 -2 -1 0 $+1$ $+2$ $+3$ $+4$ $+5$ $+6$ $+7$ $+8$ $+9$ $+10$

Interpretation

There is a bit of good news and bad news about our worseness/wellness continuum. The good news is that wellness does not really stop at plus 10; we would go broke trying to buy enough paper to spread the scale far beyond the margins to the plus thousands that are probably achievable if we genuinely work at wellness over time. Of course, you can guess the bad news going in the other direction!

Earlier, we asked you to identify any attitudes or thoughts that constitute obstacles to wellness for you. A large part of making successful changes is believing in yourself—in your potential, your ability and your resolve. Such faith isn't always easy to come by. You may be carrying messages, voices from your past that may be saying you are unworthy, undeserving, or incapable of leading a happier life. You may also have a track record of failures which colors your estimation of your potential for success in this effort. How many times have you tried to lose weight, drink less, exercise more . . . only to encounter failure down the road?

We have no magic wand to instantly dispel these unwanted thoughts and images. Chances are pretty good that they will arise, from time to time, throughout your life. Unfortunately, they're a part of who you are. For now, we would like to provide you with an opportunity to plant the seed of a more valuable image in your mind's eye: the image of who you really are when you are rid of this excess baggage.

We will be leading you through a simple visualization exercise. Visualizations are one method of nurturing your ability to change. They are a picture of your desired state. If you have never done a visualization exercise, be aware that they take a bit of getting used to. It may be helpful to have a friend read the exercise aloud to you. Soft, soothing music can assist you in relaxing, a prerequisite for visualization. Visualizations don't work for everyone, so if you find you are just not getting into it, don't worry. You'll gain something even by reading the following section. Let's begin.

Being the Best You Can Be

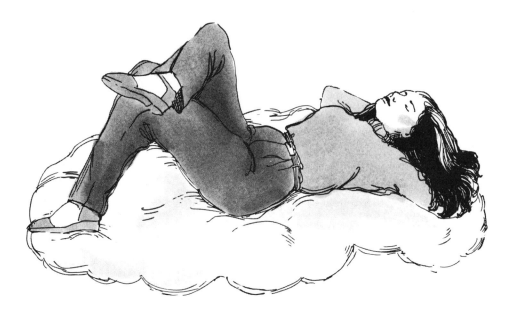

Select a five-minute period in the course of your day when you will be free of distractions and interruptions. Find a quiet spot where you can either sit comfortably in an upright position or lie on your back. Remove any restrictive jewelry or clothing, such as glasses, shoes, watches, etc.

For these five minutes, give yourself total, unfettered permission to relax completely. During this time span, there is nothing else you need to do. Everything can wait.

Close your eyes and take a deep, full inhalation. Hold your breath for a count of three, then let it out with a long sigh. Repeat this three times. Now simply allow your breath to come and go effortlessly on its own.

Imagine a warm, heavy sensation beginning in your toes and slowly moving upward into your ankles, calves, knees and thighs. Feel the warmth now penetrate your buttocks and lower back. With the next breath let all tension leave the chest, arms and hands. Imagine a warm, soothing blanket draped around your shoulders removing any traces of tightness or stiffness. Now completely relax the forehead, eye muscles, mouth and jaw. Let your tongue roll freely in your mouth.

With the next three breaths, release any tension remaining in your body.

Picture, in your mind's eye, your favorite nature spot. It can be a beach, meadow, a mountaintop, a stream, or any place which has meaning for you and in which you feel very peaceful. Imagine, in detail, all the special things about your favorite place—the colors, smells, textures, sights and sounds. It feels so good to be there.

Now imagine yourself in your favorite spot. Take a look at yourself. Note the ease and comfort in this special spot; you are filled with a sense of confidence.

Just be in this place for the remaining minutes of your relaxation break. Enjoy the imagery or visual details you have created and the physical calm and quiet of your centered body.

Now think of a time earlier in life when you were at the apex of well-being. Recall a period in either recent or distant time when you felt fully alive, joyous, and high on your natural powers and innate gifts. Envision the little things about yourself—your skin tone, the bounce in your step, the sparkle in your eyes, the comfort and ease that permeated your thoughts and actions. Re-experience for a few moments the sense of power and freedom you owned during those splendid interludes of enhanced functioning. Just smile. Enjoy a minute or so of pleasure recalling the *real* you, the person you are at your best.

Why hold back, why settle for less? Be the best you can be.

If it feels so good in memory, imagine the rewards of reaching these heights in the present. You can do it.

Now, keeping this image in mind, slowly allow your body to awaken. You feel refreshed, comfortable, and calm.

Interpretation

Visualizations provide an opportunity to populate your mind with positive and joyful self-images. When you do a visualization like this even for just a few minutes, you also reverse all the effects of the stress response: your heart rate slows, blood pressure falls, muscle reactions diminish, hormonal secretions change, and so on. This physical state which you have brought about through visualization is much more than what we normally call health, that state of "not being sick."

Quiet moments like these allow an inner voice to surface. They allow you to become acquainted with a benevolent force within you. Call it what you will—a guardian, an inner spirit, a friendly witness (your term: _____)—this inner voice is an ever-present testimony to your ability to reach your desired goals.

The best visualizations are those unique to your own experience. Use our exercise as a model for your own—and then build it into your reality with affirmations, visual cues, and rewards. Here is a vignette of how a real person employed some of these techniques in personal wellness planning.

Sherry Casteman of Miami is a public relations executive in her early thirties. She is busy in community life, athletic, a patron of the arts, and otherwise active—in addition to being a mother and a career woman. Last winter, Sherry decided to lose weight—specifically, ten pounds in three months—without restricting her eating pattern or dramatically escalating her overall activity level.

Sherry created a visualization of herself cross-country skiing on the spectacular Rocky Mountain slopes at Vail, Colorado. For 15 minutes every day, Sherry would put aside all cares and concerns, find a quiet space in her home, play some favorite Beethoven or Vivaldi, and visualize. Sherry liked to focus on the mood of the experience, the sounds of skiis sliding through the deep snow, the sensation of these treasured adventures. After about ten minutes of such imagery, Sherry would repeat a simple affirmation ("I am enjoying the attractiveness and vigor of my slim and healthy body."). Besides the visualization, Sherry reinforced her resolve by a variety of environmental cues (e.g., notes of encouragement pinned on the refrigerator and bulletin board, a slightly-too-small bikini hung in an obvious location, and similar reminders of her goal). "Effortlessly" Sherry managed to lose her unwanted pounds in two months. Her latest goal? An offer from *Playboy*—seeking her advice on a promotional campaign, of course.

Surveying Your Resources

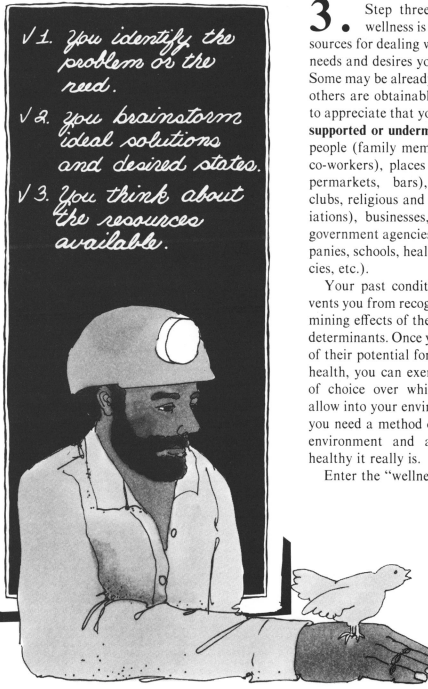

√ 1. You identify the problem or the need.

√ 2. You brainstorm ideal solutions and desired states.

√ 3. You think about the resources available.

3. Step three in planning for wellness is to survey your resources for dealing with the problems, needs and desires you have identified. Some may be already available to you, others are obtainable. First you need to appreciate that your health may be **supported or undermined** by a host of people (family members, friends and co-workers), places (restaurants, supermarkets, bars), groups (social clubs, religious and recreational affiliations), businesses, institutions and government agencies (insurance companies, schools, health planning agencies, etc.).

Your past conditioning often prevents you from recognizing the undermining effects of these environmental determinants. Once you become aware of their potential for influencing your health, you can exercise a great deal of choice over which elements you allow into your environment. But first you need a method of surveying your environment and ascertaining how healthy it really is.

Enter the "wellness canary."

The "Wellness Canary" Exercise

Not long ago, when coal mining lacked the sophisticated technology now in use to detect the presence of toxic methane gases, live canaries were taken into the mines. Canaries, it was known, are even more susceptible to the deadly but undetectable effects of methane gases than are humans. Throughout the work period, the men would keep a careful watch on the movements of the birds. When the canaries dropped dead, the miners knew it was time to make tracks—*muy pronto*—out of the mine, or in a few more minutes they, too, would join the canaries on Boot Hill.

You can use the same technique today in your quest for wellness. Instead of live canaries (too expensive), coal mines (too dirty), and sudden death (too dramatic), a few substitutions are in order.

The goal of this exercise is to identify the "methane gases" in your environment that can kill or cripple your ability to live a wellness lifestyle. Your environments are probably not coal mines; they are more likely to be high-rise buildings, school rooms, medical centers, homes in the suburbs, apartments, or combinations and/or variations of settings such as these. Because we are affected by so many different environments, there are times when we could profit from having a canary along to know whether a given environment is becoming hazardous to our health. The Wellness Canary exercise is a way to protect yourself by learning more about the kinds of environments of which you are a part, and about their effects on you.

These different environments can be seen as different "cultures." When people come together in groups, they form cultures, each with its own norms, or accepted values and expectations. Within that culture, there are tremendous pressures to conform to these values and expectations, or normal ways (norms) of doing things. Norms, usually unspoken and followed automatically without debating or otherwise thinking about them, enable us to know how to dress, speak, eat, and so on.

For the most part, these norms are innocuous; they have no influence on our health-related habits. But while there is a relatively small number of norms which *adversely* affect our lifestyles, there is an even smaller number which *positively* affect our lifestyles. Thus, we inadvertently find ourselves in a number of situations unfriendly to our health.

The challenge you face in this Wellness Canary exercise is to identify the good and not-so-good norms in a few of the cultures of which you are a part.

The exercise is quite simple: After each of the following questions just check "Yes" or "No" in the space at the right. Once you complete the exercise, we will tell you how to examine your canary to see what kind of condition it is in.

Self-Responsibility

1. At work, home and play, persons with whom you most closely associate do not smoke or drink excessively, nor are they indifferent to those who do.

   Yes _____ No _____

2. People who ride in the front seat of your automobile automatically buckle-up (as you do); if someone forgets, you do not feel embarrassed or otherwise hesitant to ask him or her to do so before driving.

   Yes _____ No _____

3. You are aware of the continuous campaign by the alcohol and tobacco producers to associate their products with the good life, beauty, youth, success, happiness, sex and so on. On occasion, you point out this trickery and fraudulent promise to young people in your care or to others who are impressionable and open to hearing a brief commentary on the seductiveness of slick advertising.

   Yes _____ No _____

4. Neither you nor your friends use recreational drugs, nor would you be supportive or accepting of others who do.

   Yes _____ No _____

5. Members of your family have been taught how to deal with minor medical emergencies; self-care is a valued skill.

   Yes _____ No _____

Nutritional Awareness

6. At your work, home and play, there is a conscious appreciation for the need to go out of the way to limit the intake of excess fat, salt, caffeine, cholesterol, refined flours and sugars, and highly processed foods.

   Yes _____ No _____

7. When you dine with friends you expect to be served whole and nutritious foods. Your friends expect the same from you.

   Yes _____ No _____

8. The school and company cafeterias which you, your children, and your friends patronize are health-conscious establishments, pleasant in mood, free of pop- and candy-vending machines, and imaginative in the range of fresh and nutritious foods served.

   Yes _____ No _____

9. There are plenty of restaurants in your area where you can enjoy nutritious and delicious foods in a smoke-free atmosphere.

Yes _____ No _____

10. You recognize that social pressures encourage rich desserts after lunch and dinner, alcohol as part of celebrations, and overindulgence in general. Fortunately, most of the people you know support each other in having fun without such departures from good health habits.

Yes _____ No _____

Physical Fitness

11. You look on exercise as a treasured time of the day. Other things (meals, travel, weather, mechanical failures, business obligations, doctor appointments, social upheavals, acts of God, and the like) may have to be postponed or endured, but almost nothing is given precedence over the daily 30- to 60-minute fitness break.

Yes _____ No _____

12. You belong to a club, group, and/or association of some kind (a jogging group, membership in a tennis club, etc.) where like-minded folks exercise with you and support the pursuit of whatever athletic habit(s) you enjoy on a regular basis.

Yes _____ No _____

13. You, your children, and/or friends look upon exercise as a pleasure, not a grind.

Yes _____ No _____

14. Whenever possible, you use stairs rather than elevators/escalators, park far enough from the office/plant to get a bit of extra exercise, and otherwise walk rather than drive.

Yes _____ No _____

15. Relatively few of your associates, relatives, playmates, and others close to you (particularly immediate family members) are sedentary—and not motivated to do something constructive about it.

Yes _____ No _____

Stress Awareness and Management

16. At your home, work and play, it is expected that people will take time to quiet themselves, to get centered and balanced, in situations of potential stress buildups.

Yes _____ No _____

17. Relaxation breaks are part of your day. At a minimum, you are able to close off the stimuli around you for brief respite when you sense the need to do so.

Yes _____ No _____

18. Your friends, children, and/or close associates decline to take on more responsibility than is reasonable for them to assume. In other words, you and those around you are able to acknowledge limits, to protect the rounded, or holistic, quality of your lives, and to express vulnerability to excessive stress loads.

Yes _____ No _____

19. In your life, there is a general understanding of the fact that stress is an essential part of life, and that how people respond to events and circumstances in their daily routines determines whether they feel drained or energized.

Yes _____ No _____

20. When possible, you talk with others about the stress phenomenon and mention something about the way stress works. Perhaps you have shown someone how to do a simple breathing or quieting exercise, or a mood calming/visualization/or imagery technique.

Yes _____ No _____

Environmental Sensitivity

21. At your home, work and play, there is an openness to discussing what it means to be a healthy person. You, your children, your mate, or close friends and associates could talk comfortably about your pictures of optimal well-being from a psychological or spiritual point of view.

Yes _____ No _____

22. You believe you have the right to ban smoking in your own home. You would not be embarrassed to post signs to this effect, and to gracefully ask relatives, friends or hired help to refrain from smoking indoors.

Yes _____ No _____

23. It is easy for you to live a wellness lifestyle given that so many others seem to be similarly oriented.

Yes _____ No _____

24. You are confident that your working environment is not a threat to your physical well-being.

Yes _____ No _____

25. Some of your friends are vigilant about the dangers of everyday toxins, such as are found in air freshners, insecticides, cleaning solvents, adhesives, fire-retardants, maintenance fluids, plasticizers, fluorescent lighting, TV, x-rays, microwaves, and asbestos, formaldehyde, and other harmful substances in carpets/furniture/and drapes.

Yes _____ No _____

Interpretation

The assessment of your environment for wellness is complete. This exercise tells you if you are supported or hindered by your cultures and the norms and values they encourage and support. All you need now is to add up your "yes" responses and you will have a measure of the quality of the environment in which your wellness canary—and you—are living.

Please place a check underneath the bird below which most closely corresponds to how your wellness canary must look, given the environment it has to contend with. Better yet, color it in hues and tones appropriate to the situation.

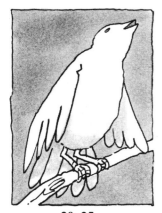

20–25
Magnifique!

This wellness canary will prosper—and so will you. Congratulations.

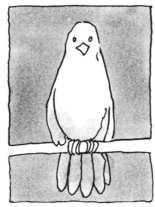

16–19
Good Quality Space

With a little extra effort, this bird should enjoy a normal life.

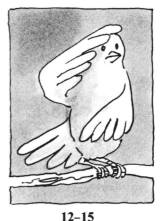

12–15
Borderline Situation

Things could go either way. Keep a close watch on the canary—and be ready to vacate the premises at a moment's notice.

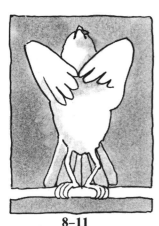

8–11
Hazardous

The yellow canary is turning green. Do something. Split at once—or fumigate the joint.

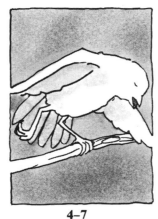

4–7
Severe Toxicity

Administer CPR—rush the poor creature to the nearest Wellness Center.

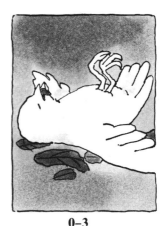

0–3
Red Alert Disaster

The canary is close to death. Try open heart massage—anything! Take action!

Conclusion

This wellness canary exercise can warn you of debilitating toxins in your environment. It can help you perceive effects which are barely noticeable until it is too late. It can alert you to a build-up of toxins from the different cultures you participate in. But the exercise can do more than warn you of the downside risks or "worseness" characteristics of what is; it can also raise your awareness of wellness and what can be. It is loaded with tips for prosperity as well as survival.

So do not feel discouraged if your canary looks a bit pale at this point. You have already gained a lot of ideas just by thinking about your environment at home, work, and play. Now you have a sense of the norms and expectations that prevail, and a pretty good idea of whether they do or do not support a wellness lifestyle.

Now it is time to do something about it. We have some ideas which we will share with you in the discussions and exercises to come. Stay loose.

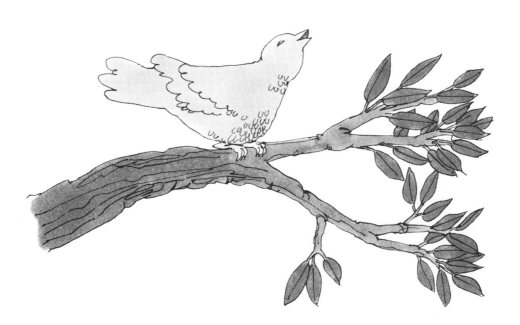

Making Choices

√ 1. You identify the problem or the need.

√ 2. You brainstorm ideal solutions and desired states.

√ 3. You think about the resources available.

√ 4. You make a choice.

4. Throughout this workbook as you *decide* to read, *decide* to think and reflect, *decide* to write or complete an exercise—you are making choices. There is nothing really special in that. You make literally thousands of choices each day.

Because your decision to enrich yourself by pursuing a wellness program is so closely tied to your choice-making process, it will be useful for you to take a moment to examine the way you make decisions. The following exercise will help you take a deeper look at your approach to "choosing."

These open-ended questions should get you in the proper mood for assessing this important phase of wellness planning. Just fill in the blanks.

• The hardest kind of choice for me to make is _____

_____

_____

_____

_____

_____

_____

_____

• The easiest kind of choice for me to make is _____

_____

_____

_____

_____

• I feel best about my choices when _____

_____

_____

_____

• If I could pick someone else to make all my choices for me for one day, I would select _____

_____

Now think about a recent decision to buy something (anything—an article of clothing, a newspaper, a sandwich). What factors prompted you to choose as you did? Specifically, did any of the following issues influence your decision?

1. Cost to you—in terms of time, money and energy
2. Quality of the item—its durability and appearance
3. Potential impact—short-term vs. long-term consequences
4. Immediate vs. long-term gratification
5. Ease or difficulty of making the choice

As you can see, each choice you make is directed by a given need or combination of needs. Sometimes you are consciously aware of the need or needs that determine your choice; other times the need can be unearthed only through deeper probing.

In making choices, you must often reconcile conflicting messages. Part of you seems to be saying one thing, part of you another. How do you know when a choice is *appropriate* (right) for you?

Think back to a recent decision you made which you now feel was wrong. In a few sentences, jot down the key elements involved in this incident.

Better yet, relate the event to a friend. _____

_____

_____

_____

Can you recall the different messages you were getting at the time you made this decision?

Part of me said _____

_____

_____

_____

while another part of me said _____

_____

_____

_____

What tipped the balance? One need took precedence over the other.

In retrospect, can you identify whether the "right" choice might have been known all along, known by the part of you which lost the debate? Was the right choice part of the message of a small inner voice? Making successful choices involves a knowledge of your innermost needs, a knowledge of the messages which continually come in from your own personal seat of wisdom. Knowing how to translate that inner voice is a reflection of your awareness of the real you. What are your purposes, values, and commitments? Later on, you will have a chance to test yourself on these issues. Since the real decision power is wielded by your purposes, values, and commitments, it makes sense to know what they are.

For now, however, we want you to make some goal-setting decisions.

Creating a Plan

√ 1. You identify the problem or the need.

√ 2. You brainstorm ideal solutions and desired states.

√ 3. You think about the resources available.

√ 4. You make a choice.

√ 5. You create a plan.

5. You have identified the problems/needs, brainstormed ideal solutions and desired states, thought about resources, and contemplated choices and options.

Now it is time for your personal two-month wellness plan.

Why two months?

A Two-Month Plan

We recommend two months for several reasons. Commitment is essential, and any lesser period does not seem sufficient to demonstrate commitment. Secondly, you need to chart your progress. It takes at least eight weeks to establish patterns which will reinforce and sustain you, which will show up on your graphs, and which will give you evidence of your ability to succeed. You need enough time to achieve some short-term rewards. Instead of establishing a goal that requires several months (e.g., loss of 30 pounds), build in a series of mini-rewards achievable within your two-month plan. Rewards do not have to be expensive or dramatic (e.g., a Carribean cruise); dinner at a special restaurant, a walk on the beach, a day off work, a new tie, and similar niceties are just as effective. We think of these moments as celebration times.

Setting Goals

Regardless of where you start, you must set a realistic and obtainable goal for yourself, one which you can reach with a modest amount of effort. The casual "wing-it" technique that serves so well for routine functions does not work as effectively for lifestyle programming. Changing our lifestyle requires conscious goal-setting.

There are at least eight areas of life which should be considered in organizing a complete personal wellness plan. (There are others, of course, but these will do for openers.) The areas are shown on the following diagram:

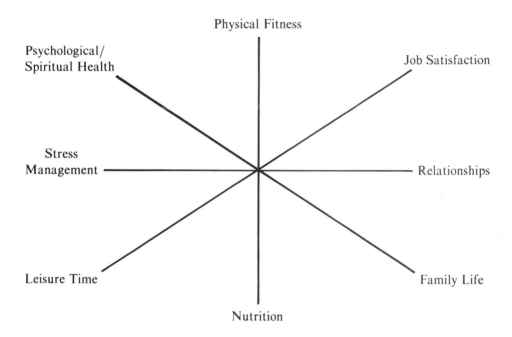

Now consider one or more of the eight areas above and take five minutes to list the goals you would like to achieve over the next two months. Please use a pencil for this exercise:

MY GOALS:

Physical Fitness: _____

_____

_____

Job Satisfaction: _____

_____

_____

Relationships: _____

_____

_____

Family Life: _____

_____

_____

Nutrition: _____

_____

_____

Leisure Time: _____

_____

_____

Stress Management: _____

_____

_____

Psychological/Spiritual Health: _____

_____

_____

You could, of course, try to change everything at once. In our experience, we have found that it is best to begin by concentrating on just one or two areas for the first two months. Leave the other areas for a time when you have already mastered the rudiments of lifestyle change.

Just in Case: You may have skipped writing your responses to the exercises so far. Not putting your reactions in written form is a mistake. Goal statements can only motivate you if you have your intentions in front of you, written out. To make it easier, you can use the forms we have provided for your use in the back of the book.

Let's look at these goals and determine whether they will serve your good intentions or undermine them.

There are five characteristics of effective goals. Examine your goal statements to see how each measures up to the following standards.

1. **Translate goals and behaviors into specific terms.** Instead of "I would like to improve my health," be specific. How about: "I will lose 10 pounds by monitoring my food intake and beginning a jogging program."

2. **Add a measurement component.** What will it take to achieve the goal? How will you know when you are ready? In the example above, you could weigh yourself weekly, calculate daily calorie intake, and log the number of minutes you jog each day. Measurement components are best when checkpoints for progress are built in. Intermediate and short-range sub-goals can be helpful.

3. Identify a **time schedule** for goal achievement. Pick a date for accomplishing your feat. How about this: "I will weigh 180 pounds by my birthday," or "Next January 1, I will be running five miles four times a week."

4. Make sure your goal is **realistic,** but also **challenging.** A goal should present a challenge that, with dedication and perseverance, can probably be realized. The prospects for accomplishing it should be favorable. Avoid goals that are too easy or too challenging (e.g., "I will lose 30 pounds this month" may be a case of attempting too much, too soon).

5. Goals should always be **in writing.** Seeing your goal statements on paper strengthens your commitment to their pursuit. It serves as a reminder of what you have undertaken and helps you think of ways to progress.

Additional steps beyond these five basics can help, too. Posting goal statements in conspicuous locations is one technique that will help you keep your goals in focus. Another is to visualize yourself in the act of celebrating goal achievements. Concentrate on the pleasures and satisfactions; revel in the glorious sense of quiet confidence that such completion affords. Phrase goals in a declarative rather than hopeful way (i.e., "I will . . ." is preferred to "I would like . . ."). Try to establish checkpoints for evaluating progress along the way, which you can check off as you near the target for accomplishing the overall goal(s).

Interpretation

Now look back at the goals you have listed. Rewrite each goal so that it is specific, measurable, time-phrased, and realistic. (Do not worry if they require drastic revision. After all, you played our game without knowing the rules!)

All clearly met the fifth measure (that goals be committed to paper); how about the other effectiveness criteria?

It sometimes happens that, in writing goals, you think of aims that you would like to pursue, accomplish, or obtain that you had not realized were so important in your value scheme. Now that you know what you want, need and deserve, it is time to select the activities which will help you realize your goals. Carrying out the plan requires not only that you do what you decided to do, but also that you build in support for maintaining your chosen course of action.

Carrying Out the Plan

√ 1. *You identify the problem or the need.*

√ 2. *You brainstorm ideal solutions and desired states.*

√ 3. *You think about the resources available.*

√ 4. *You make a choice.*

√ 5. *You create a plan.*

√ 6. *You carry out the plan and develop support for maintaining it.*

6. Now is the time to use your creative brainstorming ability. The activities you select in this section can go a long way toward supporting your good intentions. Do not be afraid to use a little imagination, to build in incentives or gentle penalties (like contributing $20 to one of the predatory tobacco companies, if you stray from the non-smoking path), or to get your friends and family involved.

Now is the time to utilize your creative abilities and capitalize upon your past experiences. There are undoubtedly an infinitive number of ways for you to reach your goal. The challenge is to select activities which you enjoy and are likely to participate in over the eight week period.

Here are some examples of real life goal-supporting activities. Pay more attention to the format than the content; your goals and activities will naturally be quite different from this illustration.

Goal Supportive Activity Commitments

Goal: Physical Fitness

Goal Statement: I will work up to exercising six times weekly for thirty minutes per session over the next two months.

Goal Supportive Activity Commitments:

- I will sign up for a yoga class at the Y.
- I will keep an exercise log.
- I will buy a new warm-up suit.
- I will put my favorite picture of myself (when trim) on the refrigerator.

Goal: Stress Management

Goal Statement: I will learn two stress management techniques by July 1.

Goal Supportive Activity Commitments:

- I will read two books on the subject within five days.
- I will buy a relaxation tape, and practice every morning for 15 minutes.
- I will park my car five blocks from work and use the walk at the end of my work day as time to unwind.

Goal: Family Life

Goal Statement: I will spend an average of eight hours each week with my two children in adventure activities for the remainder of this year.

Goal Supportive Activity Commitments:

- I will sign up for a family membership in the science museum.
- I will put aside an hour every morning for reading to and with the children.
- I will visit with the teachers to get new ideas on topics of interest.

Goal: Relationships

Goal Statement: I will improve my relationship with my in-laws to the point that I will enjoy their company at next year's reunion.

Goal Supportive Activity Commitments:

- I will try to be more tolerant of their messy habits.
- I will be more gracious when they arrive unannounced for dinner.
- I will try to remember that Uncle Harry is just being himself when he spits.

Goal: Job Satisfaction

Goal Statement: I will immediately redesign my work environment to support my wellness program.

Goal Supportive Activity Commitments:

- I will ask my wellness-oriented friends to help me plan needed changes.
- I will place the motto "I am *not* the target" in a prominent spot on my desk.
- I will share my feelings with co-workers who smoke and ask them if I might be of assistance in helping them stop smoking.
- I will contribute a nutritious whole grain casserole to each celebration (i.e., birthdays, retirement, marriage) this month.

Goal: Leisure Time

Goal Statement: I will take up sailing this summer.

Goal Supportive Activity Commitments:

- I will register for a sailing course at the local community college.
- I will let my beard grow so I look like an "old salt."
- I will try to converse more with those people at work who are interested in sailing.
- I will subscribe to a sailing magazine.

Hopefully, these examples will provide you with the necessary inspiration to create a workable wellness plan.

Now turn to the worksheets in the back of the book and complete the activity statements for each goal you have selected. When you finish this, return for a contract signing ceremony!

There is another skill which you will need to ensure that your commitment to your goal remains steadfast. It is called contracting.

The Contract Exercise

A contract can be much more than "an enforceable agreement or covenant," as defined in a dictionary. It can be an understanding that serves to make a given matter clear, concise, and direct. All of us enter into informal contracts nearly every day (e.g., agreeing to meet a friend at a specific place at a given time); occasionally, we have use for contracts of a more complex variety, such as legal contracts requiring an attorney (e.g., buying a house). A contract for wellness purposes is somewhere between these extremes. It is an invaluable tool; we recommend it because it clarifies and reinforces your determination and commitment to make lifestyle changes.

Contracts for wellness are basically written agreements with yourself. As with the goal-setting process, the act of writing an agreement down makes it more real and compelling. You can build into your contract all the necessary evaluation measurements, payoffs, rewards, and support conditions which you require to keep your commitment. The contract period might be as short as a month or as long as six months.

Here is a sample "wellness contract" which you might make with yourself to stimulate action and to stay on track in carrying out your lifestyle-enhancing goals. Your task is to fill in the blanks.

A Contract Between Myself and Yours Truly

I, _____, being of sound mind and possessed of free will, do hereby commit myself to the following goals and activities for the next two months. This agreement with myself shall be in effect from _____ until _____ . (Note: This is a somewhat formal preamble. You may prefer a more contemporary, to-the-point version such as the following.)

Count me in. I want to be part of this wellness movement. I want *my* body and *my* mind to feel great! So I am taking a pledge, an agreement, a promise, and a 100-percent "I do declare" contract with good ole #1, namely, _____ , to do all the good deeds/feats/and glorified achievements noted below.

- The goals I set for myself are:

  _____

  _____

  _____

  _____

- To pursue these goals, I will perform the following activities on a regular basis. Specifically, the time set aside for each goal is as follows (Note both the goal-related activity and when it will be performed.):

  _____

  _____

  _____

  _____

- Friends who will assist me in these pursuits are:

  _____

  _____

- I realize I may sabotage my plan by:

  _____

  _____

- So I will avoid this by:

  _____

  _____

- The payoffs which I will realize by fulfilling my goals are:

  _____

  _____

  _____

Signed _____

   Witness _____

In getting started you may find that your good intentions go astray one, two, three days or weeks down the road. Mark Twain aptly described the difficulties of remaining an ex-cigarette smoker when he declared that "stopping smoking was easy . . . I've done it dozens of time." You, too, can anticipate some down-times on your road to better health.

A few guidelines may prove helpful in carrying out your plan.

1. **Act upon your good intentions immediately.** Make a commitment to a wellness lifestyle—*now,* not later. An overt act of some kind (e.g., buying a pair of jogging shoes and setting a time to run with someone) helps.

2. **Knowledge gained through active participation is superior to information passively received from a convenient source.** Active participation leads to self-discovery. (Example: role-playing is better than a lecture; discussion groups are better than reading.)

3. **Whatever you choose to work on, do it at a moderate pace.** Too often, too much is attempted too soon at what is essentially an unstable time. Avoid discouragement by forming realistic expectations.

4. **Repetition and feedback are essential parts of skill-building.** Feedback should be immediate, encouraging, and centered on the behavior (for example, note calories burned by the exercise activity). Repetition and feedback build commitment.

5. **It's important to have early successes.** Success in terms of positive payoffs reinforces and strengthens motivation. External encouragement is good (compliments from others), but internal satisfactions are the most powerful. Positive returns are at the core of the wellness experience. You are more likely to grow stronger (psychologically) from the positive experience of adding something to your life than from the denial experience of giving something up (e.g., smoking).

6. **Take control of your environments.** Your environment is loaded with cues which reinforce habits and otherwise influence your choices. It makes sense to pay attention to the critical aspects of the physical spaces around you and reshape them to suit your goals. Surround your workspace with plants, meaningful pictures, baskets of fruit. Shut off the television. Get a full-length mirror.

7. **Hang around with the right people.** Have the courage to turn down an invitation for cake and coffee, alcohol, or cigarettes. Be aware of the power of modeling; it does matter if physicians smoke, if nurses are overweight, and if the staff at the wellness center (and the sponsoring hospital) are themselves committed to and working on personal wellness plans. Choosing your influences improves the prospects of being able to bring about the changes you desire.

8. **Chart your progress.** You can derive great satisfaction from keeping logs of your progress. Many activities lend themselves to graphing. A wellness chart can serve as a buffer against temporary short term setbacks.

Throughout this text we have included real life examples of wellness charts in use. When kept up over months and years these graphs can shed light on repeating behavior patterns. By sharing your record with others, you can heighten your own commitment while developing a valuable support group. At the back of this book, you will find several sheets of blank graph paper designed for chart keeping.

Not everyone needs or wants to keep charts, share progress with others, or design formal contracts. There are some "lone rangers" who rise daily to jog in solitary bliss, turn down temptations with iron-clad will, and basically appear to thrive regardless of their environment. Most people, however, require the support of others until their newly acquired lifestyle patterns become well established and capable of providing them with satisfaction.

Paying Attention to How Things Are Going and Adjusting as Necessary

√ 1. You identify the problem or the need.

√ 2. You brainstorm ideal solutions and desired states.

√ 3. You think about the resources available.

√ 4. You make a choice.

√ 5. You create a plan.

√ 6. You carry out the plan and develop support for maintaining it.

√ 7. You pay attention to how things are going and adjust as necessary.

7. There is no such thing as a sure fire plan. All planning efforts have a built-in measure of trial and error. Carrying out new ideas requires paying careful attention to how things are going and adjusting as necessary.

So it is with planning for wellness. You will need to carefully monitor the results of your health efforts over time to determine what parts of your program should be reinforced, redesigned, or discarded.

There is in all of us a "preprogrammed" tendency to stay with old habits of attitude and behavior which could undermine the best of plans. As you embark upon your personal wellness plan, be aware of the "worseness" robot that might be lurking somewhere within you—below the surface of consciousness.

Urges, Associations and Habits

Everyone is familiar with robots. They appear in science fiction. They are part of modern culture. They play an important role in industry.

But robots play a role that few of us ever think about, an even more influential role. In this *secret* role, robots affect our health and our prospects for pursuing a wellness lifestyle.

Robots, you see, have been installed in all of us. The robot in each of us is, quite simply, the layer upon layer of beliefs, feelings, and behaviors which we do not think about any more. These layers are automatic, unquestioned, and taken for granted. And our robot makes decisions, some of which are not so good—from a wellness perspective.

The Robot Phenomenon

A great deal of our behavior, perhaps 90 percent, is habitual. Our thoughts, feelings, and actions are often "automatic," as if we were human computers programmed to go what has to be done. We rise, dress, eat, go to work, and so on, without thinking much about it, just doing these things as we always do them.

From one point of view, this is an advantage. You would not want to have to spend a lot of time thinking about how to make the bed, which leg goes in your pants first, and so on. Our unconscious thinking and functioning, which we call our "robot," is a labor-saving, brain-conserving servant which we have trained to carry out a wide range of mechanical intentions.

However, our robot circuitry may consist of intentions and acquired patterns *not* favorable to wellness. For, in general, societal norms have not been oriented to encourage optimal health. Habitual behaviors such as smoking, excessive eating, alcohol consumption, anxiety, procrastination, and lack of organization are examples of dysfunctional actions which run on automatic pilot.

The Challenge

Your robot is designed to serve you. But it can get power hungry. It can "butt in" on your life to an excessive degree, crowding out the real you.

You can tell whether your robot is malfunctioning in this way if:

- Your robot (i.e., urges, associations, and habits) is costing you money, time and energy, and accomplishing little that is constructive in return.
- Your robot hinders your participation in enjoyable experiences.

- Your robot leads you to risk of physical harm.
- Your robot seems to irritate others.
- Your robot sometimes embarrasses you.

Like any piece of machinery, your robot deserves periodic checkups, maintenance and, for some, a drastic overhaul. There are times when robots require extensive reprogramming. Here are a few tips:

- **Watch your robot in action.** Give yourself a week or so to observe the unwanted behavior pattern. Just studying your robot in action may provide you with additional resolve.
- **Determine when your robot works,** and when it does not. In the case of overeating, determine what emotions you are experiencing, who you're with, and so on.
- **When you're ready, pull the plug,** stop the habit completely.
- **Acknowledge the fact that you'll miss your robot.** You've probably been together for years. There will be a period of loss. Accept the fact that your robot may come back to visit you, periodically.
- Finally, **send your robot back to school.** The trick is to put new "chips" in your robot. Let the robot take charge of which leg goes first and attend to other low-consciousness duties, but keep him/her away from your turf.

Use more complicated circuitry to move toward optimal health levels and ways of being. Never let the unconscious robot lead you to boredom, apathy, and satisfaction with "normal" life. Stay out of the "robot rut."

Beyond the Plan

Evaluation is as important as any other part of this seven-stage effort. You need to look at what's working and not working for you so you can replan if necessary and celebrate if not. But keep one principle in mind when assessing your results: *change is a gradual process.* Do not be too hard on yourself. Any improvement is worth self-praise and reinforcement. In fact, behavior change is more lasting if it takes place slowly, over time, so that it can be integrated into your daily life.

Journal-keeping, logbooks, or diaries of any kind will assist your personal wellness planning. Making a few practice plans and testing the process for a week or so will help you to be inventive and comfortable with wellness planning.

To assess progress, ask yourself a few questions:

- Did I work on each goal and goal-supportive activity listed in my contract?
- Did I do it as often and as long as planned?

- How did I feel when I did (or did not) do it?
- Did I enlist support from others?
- Did I reward myself adequately?
- In general, was my personal wellness plan realistic, or did I try too much too soon?
- Was I sufficiently committed to the program?
- What do I want to do next?
- How can I change the plan to make it work better?
- Was my robot under control?

To conclude this section, we thought you might be interested in a few bits and pieces of personal wellness plans developed by our students and friends.

PERSONAL WELLNESS PLAN
OF LINDA GOODRICH
San Francisco, Calif.

GOALS FOR LEISURE TIME

GOAL I: I will go dancing once a week.

Supportive Activity Commitments:

- I will ask people that I meet if they go dancing and invite myself along (in a polite way, of course)
- I will buy clothing that is fun to wear when dancing
- I will research out places that have good bands, and or recorded music
- I will tell my family that this is what I intend to do.

GOAL II: I will treat myself to one weekend away every two months.
Supportive Activities:

- I will put money away in a separate account
- I will cross out one weekend on my calendar
- I will plan at least 6 different places to go

A Contract Between Myself and Yours Truly

I, Linda Goodrich, being of sound mind and body and possessed of free will, do hereby commit myself to the following goals and activities for the next two months. This agreement with myself shall be in effect from January 2 until March 1. The goals that I set for myself are:

Payoffs: I will look a lot more sexy and beautiful
          I will feel more alive
          I will have more fun

SIGNED ___*Linda Goodrich*___ DATE _____
WITNESS ___*Leslie Kaplon*___

PERSONAL WELLNESS PLAN
OF ROBERT NEUTEBOOM
San Francisco, Calif.

I, Robert H. Neuteboom, being of sound mind and possessed of free will, do hereby commit myself to the following goals and activities for the next two months. This agreement with myself shall be in effect from March 1 until May 1.

The goals I set for family life are:

1. I will spend at least two hours each week with each child doing things they want to do.
2. I will devote at least one night a week to my wife for enhancement of our relationship.
3. I will promote family physical fitness beginning January 4.

The payoffs which I will realize by fulfilling my goals are:

1. I will feel better.
2. I will be happier.
3. I will look better.
4. I will be a healthier person.
5. I will become closer to my children.

6. I will develop a better relationship with my wife.
7. I will have healthier children.

To pursue these goals, I will perform the following activities on a regular basis. Specifically, the time set aside for each goal is as follows:

1. Each Sunday evening at 5:30pm I will discuss the time the kids and I will spend together during the coming week.
2. Each Friday evening from 7:00pm to 12:00pm will be my wife's and my time together.
3. I will eat at the same time each day as established by the family at Family Home Evening.
4. At least three evenings a week the family will exercise for 30 minutes together, this to be determined at the weekly Family Home Evening.

Friends who will assist me in these pursuits are:

1. Mary Lou
2. Kelli
3. Kim
4. Kari
5. Erin
6. Jay

I know I will have reached my goals when the following conditions prevail:

1. My family does things together.
2. My wife and I are able to get away without feeling guilty that the kids are home without us.
3. I know all the children's stories by heart and can build anything out of blocks blindfolded.

I realize I might sabotage my plan by:

1. Getting too busy to spend time with the wife and kids.

So I plan to avoid this by:

1. Organizing my time to make the best use of what is available for me and the family.

Chapter

3

Wellness Skills

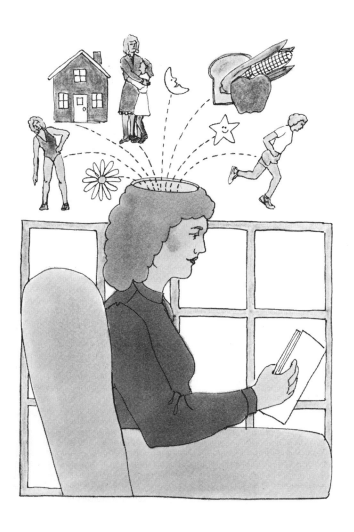

There are a number of qualities that mark success in any field. These include personal charm, a knowledge of systems, good instincts, the right environment, "inside" connections, good luck, and perseverance. There is one other quality that is more important in some professions—say brain surgery and ice skating—than in others such as politics and used car sales (though it counts there also). That quality is, of course, skill. Not just basic competence, but genuine advanced capability based on knowledge and technique.

Skill development counts a great deal in planning for wellness. It is immensely useful to have the blessings of a favorable constitution, a supportive environment, a terrific personality, and all the other qualities noted above.

But, as with brain surgery and most everything else, you will go farthest toward realizing your best potential—and savoring the journey—if you have the skills. This section is devoted to some of the rudiments of wellness skills in the areas of physical fitness, nutritional awareness, and stress management.

Physical Fitness: A Direct Line to a Wellness Lifestyle

If all five wellness dimensions are equally important but self-responsibility is **more** equal, then all dimensions also provide direct paths to a wellness lifestyle but the fitness path is **more** direct! Fitness activities provide near-immediate benefits, both physical and psychological. The physical benefits include all that goes with looking good and being sexier and feeling great; the psychological encompass raised self-esteem, control, and direction or purpose. An *incidental* benefit of a better-than-average commitment to physical fitness principles is that you drastically reduce your exposure to the risks of degenerative disorders.

So, what is a better-than-average commitment? What are the key principles? How do you avoid the usual pitfalls and make fitness a regular part of your life?

Like the family medicine kit, knowledge concerning physical fitness should be present in every home. You do not need the training of a cardiologist or exercise physiologist to be literate about physical fitness. We would like to direct a few questions your way; if you know the answers to most of the questions, you already have the basic knowledge about fitness you need.

The Fitness Quiz

1. An ideal exercise program includes which of the following (check just one):
- ☐ **A.** endurance or aerobic activities which involve the major skeletal muscles and an elevated heart rate over a given period of time, such as 20 minutes, practiced four to six times weekly
- ☐ **B.** stretching routines
- ☐ **C.** strength-building activities
- ☐ **D.** all the above

2. Examples of aerobic exercises which best provide the beneficial effects of cardiorespiratory activity are:
- ☐ **A.** basketball, handball, squash, and tennis
- ☐ **B.** distance running, swimming, hiking and biking
- ☐ **C.** horseback riding, skiing (downhill), bowling and horseshoes

3. Sprinting for a bus (or anything else), running up three flights of stairs, and going through a parcourse (circuit training) are all examples of which type of exercise?
- ☐ **A.** aerobic or endurance
- ☐ **B.** strength-building
- ☐ **C.** flexibility
- ☐ **D.** a bit of each, but mainly strength-building
- ☐ **E.** anaerobic

4. A low resting heart rate suggests:
- ☐ **A.** good physical condition
- ☐ **B.** obesity
- ☐ **C.** lack of energy
- ☐ **D.** all the above

5. The best way to recuperate from strenuous exercises is:
- ☐ **A.** to drop over and lie still for one minute
- ☐ **B.** do deep knee bends and varied calisthenics
- ☐ **C.** do the same exercise very slowly

6. The principal benefit of daily exercise is:
- ☐ **A.** reduction of heart disease risk
- ☐ **B.** ability to "fork out" at meals with less risk of weight gain
- ☐ **C.** feel better physically and psychologically
- ☐ **D.** all of the above

7. The basic measure(s) of adequacy for exercise is (are):
☐ **A.** intensity (how hard you work), frequency (how often), and duration (how long)
☐ **B.** whether you have fun doing the exercise
☐ **C.** whether you can impress your friends and neighbors doing it

8. Spot reduction, that is, losing weight in one selected area of the body:
☐ **A.** does not work; if it did, gum chewers would have skinny faces
☐ **B.** is not a valuable substitute for cardiovascular or aerobic exercise
☐ **C.** is usually a gimmick for advertising equipment, spas, and quick fix techniques
☐ **D.** all the above

9. You can tell if a person gets too little exercise because he/she will:
☐ **A.** be peevish and morose
☐ **B.** have dark circles under the eyes
☐ **C.** have sweaty palms and a suspicious look
☐ **D.** be blind at an early age
☐ **E.** show other symptoms of self-abuse
☐ **F.** none of the above has been proven scientifically

10. Certain risks of exercise (low back pain, muscle pulls, etc.) can be minimized by:
☐ **A.** regular calisthenics
☐ **B.** cold showers or baths
☐ **C.** soaking in a hot tub
☐ **D.** slow and gentle stretching routines before and after exercise, with a few minutes' warm-up and cool-down periods

Interpretation
The best answers, in our opinion, are:
1. 2. 3. 4. 5. 6. 7. 8. 9. 10.
D   B   E   A   C   D   A   D   F   D

These questions should give you an idea of your overall knowledge in this key wellness dimension.

All of us would agree on the importance of fitness, yet how can we judge what our level of fitness is? Here is an idea.

The Watershed Exercise

Make a list of characteristics which you associate with health and well-being. Suppose you wanted to know how *healthy* you were without relying on any of the usual illness measures. What would you want to check, or to what kinds of conditions would you pay attention?

Take just five minutes and make a list. Begin. _____

_____

_____

_____

_____

Interpretation

How did you do? Were you able to define some wellness characteristics? Are you satisfied with the responses that came to mind? There are two kinds of answers to this last question.

The first is what could be called subjective. These answers might include high energy levels, enthusiastic outlook, and so on. Good skin tone and clear eyes are other subjective measures of health.

The second kind of answer could be considered objective, in the sense of being verifiable, measurable, and not likely to be misinterpreted. We call these health measures "wellness vital signs."

Most people have no idea of their wellness vital signs. You may not have listed any of these measures. However, it makes good sense to know these characteristics about your body *before* you start a wellness program. In this way, you can see clear evidence of progress as you improve. This evidence will make you feel good, strengthen your motivation, and affirm what you are otherwise just suspecting—namely, that your level of functioning is truly moving far beyond the margins of just "not being ill" toward heights of genuine excellence.

Here are the wellness vital signs and a brief note on what is significant about each.

- **Resting heart rate.** Should be less than seventy beats per minute. This rate is a condition of heart muscle strength; a well-conditioned heart pumps more oxygen-rich blood with less effort than a "normal" heart. After a few weeks of strenuous aerobic exercise, your resting rate will come down. You will be able to do more work with less effort over extended periods of time.

- **Body composition.** How much of you is fat versus lean muscle tissue is important. If male, you are fit if you have 15 percent or less fat; if female, 19 percent. Did you list body composition? Do you know what your percentage is? If not, have it checked at a YMCA or YWCA, a fitness club, wellness center, or somewhere in your area. It is an inexpensive and a *vital* thing to know. With exercise at the recommended level (see next vital sign), the composition of your body will change. You will lose fat and gain muscle tissue. At first, you may not lose weight; you may even gain a few pounds (muscle is heavier than fat). Pretty soon, however, you will notice a welcome change in this measure and in your physical appearance.

- **Training heart rate.** If you know how hard to work your body (particularly the cardiovascular system), then you are in a position to get the greatest return from your chosen exercise. There are three things to know about training heart rate: (1) what yours is, (2) how often to exercise at this level, and (3) how long to exercise at this level.

Here are some guidelines. (We encourage you to read up on this in some of the recommended books on the fitness dimension of wellness and to talk with local experts at the nearest fitness or wellness center.)

1. Your training heart rate should be 70 percent of your maximum heart rate. Start with 220, the theoretical maximum human rate. Subtract your age from 220. This gives your own actual, or at least predicted, maximum heat rate. This is the figure you use to calculate how many beats per minute you should experience to get the best effect of aerobic or cardiovascular exercise. Again, here are the numbers: 220 maximum human heart rate

   — minus your age
   = *your* predicted maximum heart rate

Let's say you are 70 (congratulations). Your maximum heart rate would be 150. Seventy percent of 150 would be 105. To get the best training effect from exercise, you should jog, swim, walk, or whatever you like to do in such a manner as to raise your heart rate to 105 beats per minute.

2. Exercise at this level of exertion every day. The evidence supports four times a week, but we say every day, if possible. If not, six days. If not, whatever you can do, as often as you can do it.

3. Exercise at your aerobic training rate for at least 20 minutes. This gives you the best benefits without diminishing returns (i.e., modest further advances for disproportionately vigorous efforts).

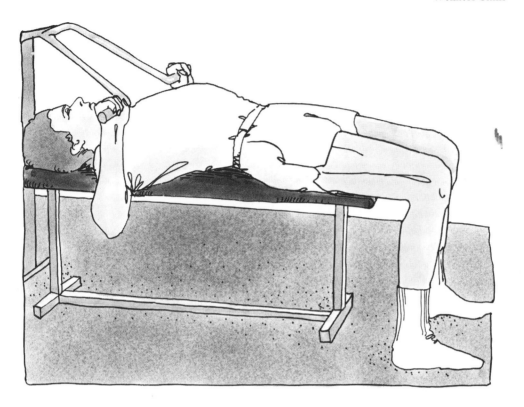

- **Another vital sign is recovery heart rate.** If you are well conditioned, your heart works better in many ways. It can return to a normal rate more quickly following vigorous exertion. (In addition, it is less likely to stop without warning, which could be embarrassing and untimely.) Here is how to check this sign: After you reach your target rate, stop. Wait one minute. Your heart rate (after one minute) should drop at least 25 beats. This is another indication of your conditioning; it will change (drop more) as you become fitter.

- **Oxygen uptake.** The better shape you're in, the more oxygen you can deliver to your body. You need a treadmill or bicycle ergometer and a tester or two to learn about this wellness vital sign. If you can afford it and have access to a place where such measures are taken, go for it. A sub-maximal test will let you know how much oxygen you can absorb and utilize. Such a test measures your system's capacity to transport oxygen from the lungs to the contracting muscles during exercise. Again, this will change as you get fitter.

- **Flexibility.** Can you touch the floor without bending your knees? Touch your toes when sitting with legs extended? There is no single measure of flexibility, but you might want to check how you do in various positions. Trunk flexion, back hyperextension, and joint range of motion are among the indicators that will change as you devote a few minutes before and after each conditioning session to these important "warm-up" periods.

- **Upper body strength.** How many chin-ups, pull-ups, or push-ups can you do? Many people can't even do one. Upper body strength can be developed readily through calisthenics, aerobic dance, swimming, and light weight training (doing 10–15 repetitions of each exercise). It's surprising how quickly even the most out-of-shape person can improve.
- **Abdominal muscle strength.** For those who sit behind a desk, weak abdominal muscles are a hazard leading to injuries and strains. Lie on your back, legs bent, with both feet on the ground—unsupported. Raise your torso. You cannot? Practice trying every day. In a few sessions, perhaps after a week or less of several attempts daily, you will. And your profile will improve.

This concludes our discussion of the wellness vital signs. All are "watershed" indicators. They let you know where you were at the beginning, and thus dramatize progress being made. While you are at it, pay attention to and enjoy your daily headpleasures, stomach delights, back strength, and ears tingling. Combine these with attention to subjective indicators, and you will be more alert to positive health. Finally, help your friends to start thinking about positive health.

Building Commitment

Along with an understanding of fitness, a better-than-average commitment implies a *daily* routine of some kind that you enjoy and value, designed to provide and sustain a state of *cardiovascular competence*. Your fitness routine is something you perform, if not daily, then at least four to six times a week, for not less than half an hour per session.

Curious about that phrase "cardiovascular competence"? Well, we just made it up. It means that your exercise activity produces the benefits for your heart and lungs that come from exercising aerobically at the necessary rate. This, in brief, is what better-than-average exercise is about.

There are **ten key principles** for achieving the near-term, as well as long-range, benefits of physical fitness. **One** is to select exercise(s) that you enjoy. Not everybody enjoys jogging. It *is* socially acceptable not to jog; it *is* possible to be fit without jogging. But you have to do something that you do enjoy that produces some of the same benefits. How about fast walking, swimming, biking, rope jumping, jazzercise, or cross-country skiing? It is possible you have convinced yourself that you do not like any of these activities. In that case, change your mind. Decide you *do* like _____ (fill in the name of an activity you just decided is great fun). Decide to invest a little time, energy, and even money to experiment with activities you have not liked for years. Commit yourself **part** of the way. Join a fitness club on a trial basis. Rent a bike for a week. Borrow a walking stick. Make your own Kung Fu robe. Sign up for several fitness classes at the local wellness center. You could be in for a pleasant surprise.

A **second** principle is to involve others, especially those who are close and important to you. For people getting started, it is true that mild discomfort (if not misery) likes company.

The **third** principle is timing. If you pick evenings after work as your exercise period, your chances of failure are higher. Studies have shown that the highest drop-out rates occur for those who try to schedule their activity for this time of day. It often happens that other demands at this time are overwhelming. In addition, you are tired and still preoccupied with the workday. Your body is home, but your head (or at least your soul) has not arrived yet. But whatever time you select, remember that you can always change your exercise schedule without giving up the commitment to exercise.

A **fourth** principle is to design a home fitness center. You do not need an olympic-sized pool, a running track, or a fully equipped weight room to have a special place in your home that reinforces and facilitates a superb state of physical fitness. It never hurts to belong to a club, gym, "Y", or other well appointed establishment, but such places are not necessarily complete, convenient, or affordable for everyone all the time. Whether you belong or not, think about the possibilities of a home fitness center.

There are three versions of such a home fitness center as we have in mind. The first is the "Everyperson" model, the second is for the "Truly Commited," and the third is the "Rolls Royce" edition.

The "Everyperson" model is where you should start if this idea appeals; it is probably suitable for 90 percent of wellness practitioners. Here is a list of what you need for making best use of this prototype:

- a room at least 6′×6′, available for part-time use as a fitness center
- a gym mat or suitable carpet for stretching
- a board that can be placed on an incline for abdominal exercises
- jump rope
- *you* need shorts, t-shirt, and sneakers
- optional: mirrors on the walls
          radio and/or tv

If this turns out to be a good thing for you and you want to escalate things a bit, then you are ready for the "Truly Commited" version of the home fitness center. Here are the requirements and options:

- everything mentioned in the "Everyperson" model above, except the sneakers and t-shirt.
- *now* you need form-fitting stretch shorts with nylon tricot fabric and poly-cotton shirts for cooling, plus lightweight running shoes with built-in orthodics
- a room at least 12′×12′ not to be used for anything else
- chin-up, pull up bar
- an assortment of free weights
- a trampoline or rebounder
- a stationary bike or ergometer
- optional: wall pulleys
            a juice bar
            stereo tape deck/record player/portable unit w/headphones
            a log in which to note your progress and achievements
            a small bookcase to keep your fitness books and magazines

If all this leaves you craving more, then you are ready for the "Rolls Royce" home fitness center. Requirements are:

- all the above, for starters, in a room at least 15′×15′
- Nautilus equipment or a multiple weight station machine
- gravity inversion boots and paraphernalia
- designer *work out* clothes
- motorized treadmill
- a Betamax-type video system with remote controls
- hot tub/jacuzzi/sauna/ or steam bath.

We do recommend consideration of the "Everyperson" approach. The whole idea is not as far out as it might have seemed a few years ago. Many major manufacturers report that home fitness center sales are their biggest markets today, whereas once they sold exclusively to figure salons, gyms, and sport clubs. Why not get in position to ride the wave of the future, ESPECIALLY if you live in a harsh climate area or do not like the idea of running around the neighborhood half naked. Have fun in your center; deck the walls with posters that conjure fantasies of athletic conquest or which recall past glories. Pin your medals on the walls, hang your ribbons from the ceiling, and spread your trophies everywhere. Do not be discouraged if you do not have any; terrific medals and trophies for the sports of your choice can be obtained real cheap at garage sales. Do not overlook the psychological aspects of your home fitness center; these recommended touches add a needed panache.

Last but not least on this point, remember that spending money does not increase your cardiovascular endurance, flexibility, or strength—exercise does that.

The **fifth** principle is to establish physical fitness goals and routines with your support group. Have each member of the group, for example, write a contract with herself/himself, and identify ways that others can help. People at work and at home can lend support to each other's fitness goals.

Share your contracts with each other—and initial your consent if you agree to help out. Take fitness outings together; make the connections between vigorous activity, enjoyment, good food, and relaxation.

Fitness activities are one of the easiest aspects of a wellness plan to develop, as the goals are easily measurable and the exercises lend themselves to charting.

Here is an example:

Terry O'Shea is a bookkeeper in Portland, Oregon. She leads a busy life while caring for her five-year-old son and busing back and forth to several freelance bookkeeping jobs. Terry established the following wellness plan:
GOAL: To lose five pounds each month by cutting my calories down to 1200 each day and getting 25 minutes of vigorous activity four times a week.
GOAL SUPPORTING ACTIVITIES:
  1. Calorie counting each day
  2. Weekly weighing
  3. Stationary bicycle
  4. Brisk walking (non-stop)
  5. New cookbook

Terry's contract included a pair of new earrings as a short-term reward upon losing five pounds (for the first month), a long-distance phone call for the second month.

On the next page is her exercise chart which she shared on a weekly basis with one of her clients who agreed to help support her efforts.

The **sixth** principle we will emphasize is to be creative in linking fitness to other parts of your life. Here is one example of what we mean: gift buying. How about if, instead of perfume and sweets and alcohol and other nefarious gift-giving on Valentine's Day, Mother's Day, birthdays, and so on, you were to give fitness gifts? There is so much from which to choose: warm-up suits, sports bags, swim suits, gift certificates to a club, favorite books, and so on. Would this not be a fine way to support those you love—and send them a nice message at the same time?

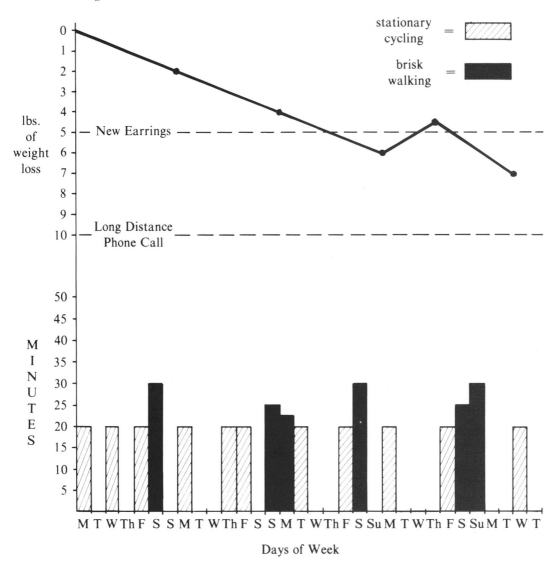

The **seventh** fitness principle is to design a balanced program. It is OK to specialize in something, but make a habit of rounding out your aerobic routine with a bit of flexibility and strength-building activity. Flexibility or stretching exercises are a quiet affair with the side-benefit of relaxation. Stretching involves slowing down and warming up by gently elongating the major skeletal muscles. It does not include any jerky movements, called ballistic movements because of their sudden, explosive manner (e.g., jumping jacks). Let gravity work for you. Use deep breathing. Give special attention to lower back stretches, the hamstrings and quadriceps, and the neck and shoulder areas. Strength-building might include abdominal tightening, light lifting, and moderate weight training. (If you embark on a program of weight training, get some supervision to start off.) All this is enjoyable in itself; it also prevents soreness and minimizes the risk of injuries or unnecessary fatigue from aerobic exercise.

The **eighth** is to know when enough is enough. Even the greats have bad days, get hurt, bored, or run down. Missing a day here and there is of no consequence to fitness or performance. Rest periods safeguard perspective, keep you from burning out, and provide opportunities for diversion. Just do not take off *too* long.

The **ninth** principle is to select a model. Whom would you like to emulate? Whose paths seem attractive? Use the model as a guide and reference, not a standard to struggle to surpass.

The **tenth** and last principle is to periodically test yourself and review both your knowledge and your progress in becoming gorgeous and *a credit to your race*. (A ridiculous phrase, but we needed something with a zing to it.)

This concludes the section on fitness skills. Enough talk and theory. Now go out and sweat.

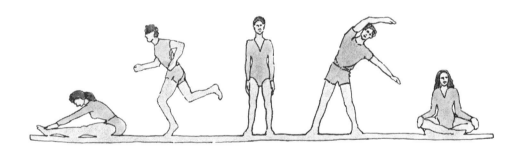

Nutrition: It's Simpler Than You Think

In Buddhism, we find a theory which explains the "twofold nature" of error. This is expressed in terms of the Near Error and the Far Error; both are believed to block the path to the goals of health and balance.

The Buddhist idea of the twofold nature of pitfalls on the path has some application to nutrition in modern life. The Near Error might be the indiscriminate wolfing down of convenience foods with little thought to their nutritional content; the Far Error might be the faddish nitpicking based on conjecture and dogma. The middle way—the one that rings true biochemically in that it provides us with building blocks for body maintenance and fuel for energy in daily life—is relatively simple. It requires, first of all, that eating be placed in the context of the whole of our life; that, in other words, we consider not just the nature of food, but the way we relate to food.

The middle way invites an emphasis on whole foods, rather than either refined goodies or supercharged supplements. It requires moderation in eating, the exercise of our natural preference for freshness and quality, and a constant attempt to bring to our table the ultimate spice: variety.

This skills section will help you assess how you relate to food, guide you in determining the quality of your diet, provide you with some facts about nutrition and, through the examples of others, show you how the Planning for Wellness System can aid in improving your food habits, losing weight and enhancing performance.

Relating to Food

When it comes to eating, we humans are creatures of habit.

Many of our eating habits are formed early in life, a gift—or handicap—from our parents. We like our peas and carrots just the way Mom used to make them. We may also eat in the same manner as our parents—slowly or quickly, quietly or in a flurry of talk and activity.

Other eating habits arise from newer life situations. That daily breakfast of coffee and a doughnut on the way to work is necessary—or so the harried worker reasons—because there are simply not enough minutes in the morning.

A peaceful meal which is followed by a short period of restful activity (let the dirty dishes sit for a while) allows the digestive tract to begin its work unimpeded.

Eating regular balanced meals of moderate size with little or no snacking in between has been found by Dr. Lester Breslow of UCLA to be one of seven common practices correlated with better health and longevity. Starting the day with a good solid breakfast is another.

We have constructed a simple self-test to help you evaluate your own eating habits. This test is designed primarily to stimulate your thinking in a number of specific areas, but it can also give you a rough idea of where you stand in the spectrum of food-related behavior.

To take this test, get out a pencil and paper and record the numerical value of each answer. You have a choice of five answers: Never (0), seldom (1), occasionally (2), frequently (3) and always (4).

How often do you:

Eat excessively when bored, depressed or nervous? _____

Use foods for reward or punishment? _____

Skip breakfast? _____

Eat foods which you know are "bad"? _____

Eat when you are not hungry? _____

Feel rushed while eating? _____

Worry or feel guilty about the number of calories in your food? _____

Eat or drink in secrecy? _____

Prefer to eat alone rather than with friends or family? _____

Go on "binges"? _____

Eat snacks shortly before retiring? _____

Eat to the point of being stuffed? _____

Eat a fast-food meal? _____

Total _____

Interpretation

If your total score was below 10, your eating habits are impeccable (and you have beaten the scores of the authors). From 10 to 16, your eating habits are "moderate and sensible"; from 17 to 25, "you could improve"; 25 to 35, "time to seriously consider some changes"; and 36 and above "out to lunch."

If your score is in the "could improve" range or higher, you may want to use the test as a tool for making a few improvements in your eating habits.

Take a look at the questions which you answered "always" or "frequently." These are your real trouble spots. To begin a process of change, pick one specific area (represented by a question above) in which you would like to improve, and ignore the rest. If you always skip breakfast, snack late at night, and eat to the point of being stuffed, you have an ingrained and potentially unhealthy eating pattern that cannot be changed overnight. Focus on improvement in one area first (in this case, we would suggest starting with a regular breakfast).

Use the Planning for Wellness system to focus on individual goals that represent a partial change. Set a measurable and time-specific target for changing an eating habit, and support that target with all the elements that reinforce adherence and success.

Just so you don't think we are perfect purists, belonging to a "nobility of the well" above the level of common, ordinary folks like you, permit us to get personal for a moment. We plan, too. The fact is, we created a short-term plan for ourselves while writing this book. Writing engenders its own set of unique tensions: in addition to the pressure to be witty, factual, poetic, and comprehensive, there looms the ever-present deadline. Our reaction to all this stress was a fairly common one; we ate more, at a record pace.

Basically, we noticed that in company with friends in restaurants, we invariably found ourselves finishing dessert while others were still contemplating the menu. Though people expressed amazement at the speed by which we consumed vast portions of delectables, we really did not think too much of it—until we noticed a crowd around us one evening going OOOH and AAAAH as we sprinted through our entrée. The message that made us finally realize something should be done was the call from network television. The producer of "That's Incredible" wanted us to eat on the show.

So we talked about the problem, considered the options, and made a choice. We would slow our pace, enjoy food more, and practice what we preach.

Our goal: To slow the pace and embellish the pleasure of restaurant dining during the writing of *Planning for Wellness*. Our goal-supportive list included the following:

- We would breathe deeply after each bite of food.
- We would use but one fork at a time.

- We would say grace before each meal.
- We would wait until after we were seated before ordering.
- We would be seated during the entire meal.
- We would return the utensil to the table after each morsel.
- We would talk about something other than *Planning For Wellness*.
- We would try not to brainstorm ideas and get excited.
- We would floss and dry brush after the main course.

We wrote a list of barriers that could get in the way of our splendid intention. These included:

- We might forget.
- We might decide "the hell with it".
- We might be too hungry to comply.
- We might feel silly.
- It might be fun to appear on "That's Incredible."
- We might say there's no time.

The payoffs we wrote included:

- We will derive more nutritional benefit from our meals.
- We will enjoy our food more.
- We will choose better restaurants.
- We will no longer make our friends who dine with us nervous.
- We will be able to give lectures on the virtues of peaceful food habits.

Our contract, signed by three waitresses, a dishwasher, and the Maitre d', was as follows:

> DBA and MT, being of sound mind and body, wish to set a better example for the youth of the universe by eating slowly as well as nutritionally. We will adhere to the goal described for a period of two weeks. Signed and witnessed.

Our friends, Charles, Diane, and Robin agreed to be our support group, and observed us on ten occasions. We did achieve our goal—we could tell because we no longer entered and departed a restaurant in less than six minutes. We spent hours (and got less work done), but it was worthwhile.

In many cases, successful improvement in one area can start a chain reaction, and lead to improvement in many others. The important thing to remember is that even though eating habits are deeply ingrained, change is possible, once you become clear about which small, specific steps you should take first.

If you scored well on the relating to food habits test, before you pat yourself on the back we should point out that the test leaves out one major component of healthy eating: The nutritional quality of the food. It is theoretically possible to achieve an "impeccable" ranking while subsisting on a regular diet of potato chips and chocolate eclairs. Your food habits, therefore, are but one side of the coin. The food itself is the other.

The "What's Coming Down" Exercise

The first step toward better nutrition is a cold, hard look at what you are now eating—in nitty, gritty detail. Simply reflecting on the general direction of your diet or your philosophy of diet will not do. For a truer evaluation of the nutritional quality of your diet, we want you to keep a three-day record of everything you eat. No matter how well nourished you think you are, or how much attention you give to your diet, you will probably be surprised at the end of these days.

For these three days, do not try to alter your normal pattern in any way. Avoid or resist the temptation to look good. Simply make a record of what you consume. Unlike calorie charts, which place emphasis on the *amount* of various foods, your three-day dietary record is concerned with *quality*.

In a sequential fashion, simply list the foods you eat throughout the day, as in the example below. Be honest. This is not a test, only a means to help you evaluate the quality of your dietary intake. Feel free to take some artistic license in the margins. For example, if you believe there are certain emotional states which play a role, note them.

EXAMPLE:
Three Days in the Stomach of _____

	Food Items	**Place**	**Mood**
Day I:			
Morning	2 eggs coffee rolls milkshake	Home	Raring to go—high after a five-mile run

| Mid-day | Avocado and cheese sandwich bread spearmint tea apple | Work | Preoccupied |
| Dinner | broiled red snapper steamed broccoli spinach salad coffee | Home | Relaxed and content |

Day II

Day III

Interpretation

When you have completed your three-day record, get out a red pen or pencil. Let's take a moment to go through a breakdown of your individual diet.

1. Start by circling those foods which are rich in simple sugars.

Pop, ice cream, candies, gum, life-savers should leap out at you. Less obvious may be some of the foods which contain hidden sugars, such as tomato ketchups with approximately 29% sugar, non-dairy coffee creamers (65%), prepared salad dressings (30%), and some cereals (25%).

You know that *we* know that *we all* know the bottom line on refined sugar—it's empty calories devoid of vitamins and minerals, contributes to cavities, obesity, and the sugar blahs. How about substituting more fresh fruit for those refined goodies?

2. How much fat are you eating?

Circle all red meats and whole milk products. These items are loaded with fat and probably contribute to heart disease and stroke. Most nutritionists recommend:
- cutting down on red meats by eating more chicken, fish, and meatless meals.
- substituting low-fat for whole-milk products.

3. Where are those whole grains?

Scan your three-day record. See any brown rice, whole wheat, millet, bulgur, oats? These grains are rich sources of vitamins and minerals, protein, and complex carbohydrates, and provide bulk for the diet. Whole grains help stretch the family's food dollar. They can be served hot for breakfast, added to soups, and made into tasty casseroles.

4. Check your diet record for vegetables.

When you opt for convenience as opposed to quality in your food selections, vegetables often get relegated to a back-seat position. Raw and lightly steamed or pan-sautéed vegetables provide valuable nutrients, especially vitamins A, B, and C. Get into the habit of eating salads, and you'll soon have vegetables a mainstay in the diet.

5. Finally, what are you drinking?

How many cups of coffee, glasses of pop, drinks of wine, beer or hard stuff are you consuming each week? Each of these beverages has well-known health hazards associated with its ingestion. (If you are not familiar with the hazards, please see the nutrition section in the bibliography section at the end of the book for further details.) Herbal teas, fruit and vegetable juices, skim milk, and plain old water serve you better.

Okay, How Much Do You Really Know About Nutrition?

The subject of nutritional science is a fascinating one. It has captivated scientists, at the very least, for the last century.

Today, there is an abundance of so-called nutritional experts and gurus. Nutritional promoters promise us instant energy, weight loss, improved sexual performance, hair growth and memory if we agree to follow their regime, adhere to their program, take their workshop and/or buy their products.

Frankly, it is very easy to be confused. We believe it is important that everyone have a basic knowledge of nutritional facts. Without knowledge, you cannot make an intelligent choice or safeguard yourself from the appeals of quackery.

We have devised a simple multiple choice quiz to help you assess your knowledge of nutrition. Ready?

1. How many pounds of simple, refined sugar does the average American consume each year?

   A. 10   **B.** 48   **C.** 125   **D.** 312

2. What product is comprised of the following ingredients?
   Water, hydrogenated coconut and palm kernel oils, sugar, corn syrup, sodium caseinate, dextrose natural and artificial flavors, polysorbate 60, sorbitan monostearate, xanthan gum, guar gum, artificial color.

   A. rocket fuel   **B.** deodorant   **C.** dog food
   D. a popular topping whip

3. The fat-soluble vitamins are

   A. A, D, E and K   **B.** A, B, E, and D   **C.** C, E, and K
   D. A and B

4. How many calories must one shed to lose a pound of body fat?

   A. 150   **B.** 2000   **C.** 3500   **D.** 5000

5. Walking a mile uses how many calories?

   A. 50   **B.** 100   **C.** 500   **D.** 1000

6. Where is most of the usable protein found in an egg?

   A. shell   **B.** white   **C.** yellow

7. In the average American diet, what percentage of calories comes from fats?

   A. 10   **B.** 20   **C.** 30   **D.** 40

8. Ideally, what percentage of calories in diet should be obtained from fat?

   A. 5%   **B.** 10–25%   **C.** 45% or more

9. Regarding protein, which statement is true?

   A. You must have meat every day to get enough protein.
   B. Vegetables, beans, and grains don't have any protein in them.
   C. The best food for athletes is steak before a game.
   D. Combinations of beans and grains produce whole usable proteins which can meet our requirements for this substance.

10. Fortified whole milk provides which of the following nutrients?

    A. protein, vitamin D, calcium, fat   **B.** protein, vitamin B, iron
    C. protein, vitamin C, magnesium, zinc
    D. fat, vitamin K, selenium, chloride

If you scored between 8 and 10 correct answers, chances are you have a good scientific understanding of nutrition. For those who scored less than 8, gathering some factual knowledge about nutrition will help you make intelligent food choices for yourself and family members.

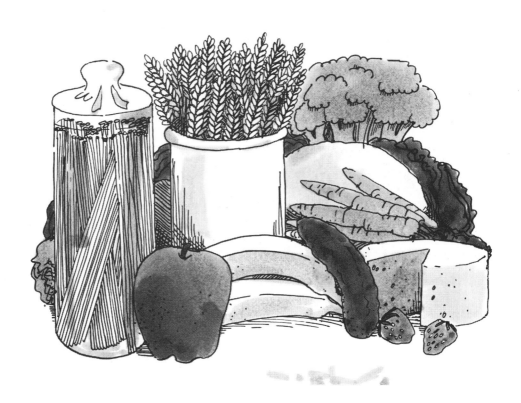

Losing Weight

Losing weight has become a national preoccupation. Approximately fifty percent of all adults are attempting to shed unwanted pounds. North Americans have become experts in the dieting game. The problem with most diets, of course, is that they are just diets. This guarantees failure. Without an exercise component, a change in food habits, awareness of adverse norms and attention to stress issues, diets will be fleeting and any changes transitory.

In order to lose weight permanently, you must change your lifestyle patterns permanently, including how, why, and what you eat.

Despite the fact that most Americans intuitively know this, fad diets, which ignore exercise and other lifestyle components, remain as popular as ever.

Inasmuch as you or your next door neighbor is probably on a diet (and will be again next year) we thought we would address this area in the skills section. The Planning for Wellness process can be used for developing greater nutritional awareness and losing extra pounds over the short term, but the real advantage of the system is that it will provide you with an effective method for maintaining weight loss in concert with other wellness advances.

Before we get into the specifics, let's cover some definitions so that we begin with the same understanding.

Overweight: This is a standard of comparison. It is based upon a set of height/weight norms developed by life insurance companies derived from correlations between morbidity and mortality. Unfortunately, these measures ignore the variables of body structure and condition. It is possible to be overweight yet neither fat nor obese. For example, a large-boned, muscular athlete may tip the scales in excess of statistical norms. Thus, he would be considered overweight. Yet when condition is factored in, he may in fact have little or no excess weight. To explore this, a few comments about fat, calories, and energy are in order.

Fat: Fat is a wonderful fuel. It is a highly concentrated, stored form of energy. When your body burns a pound of fat, 3500 calories are "liberated"—enough to fuel a 35-mile walk!

Most Americans wear too much fat. (Researchers at the University of Illinois have calculated that the national total of excess fat is in the neighborhood of 2.3 billion pounds.) Ideally our bodies should contain not more than 15 percent fat (men) or 19 percent (women); the contemporary "scores" are not even close to these ideals (*23* percent for men, *36* percent for females*).

*Gary Dalton, "Expert Opinions on Health and Medicine," *City Sports,* March, 1982, p. 8.

Calorie: A calorie is a unit of energy which is released when a substance (carbohydrate, fat or protein) is metabolized by the body. Each gram of fat contains 9 calories while carbohydrate and protein contain approximately half as much. This is why adding a small pat of butter equates in calories with consuming a large potato.

Energy: Our bodies run on glucose for fuel. It is the dollar, or unit of exchange, for energy. Glucose is obtained for body fuel from a number of sources—from the diet, from stored glycogen in the liver, from the breakdown of protein in muscles, and from the catabolism of fat. Fat bodies draw heavily upon the first three sources for energy, and experience great difficulty in "burning" fat. Why? Without regular exercise, muscles (along with our brains, the major users of fat and glucose) adapt to a pattern of consuming an extremely low amount of fat. The muscles lose interest in consuming fat calories. Therefore, the enzymes and cellular reactions responsible for providing energy operate at a very low level. Consequently, fewer calories are burned—and you get to keep the savings. In this case, that's not a good deal.

Regular exercise stimulates the production of calorie-consuming enzymes. Even as little as twenty minutes of moderate activity daily will promote these healthy changes.

Instant Success: Most cases of instant success are followed by later cases of sudden failure. The longer weight loss takes, the longer the changes are likely to last. A modest, realistic pace for weight loss is one to two pounds a week.

Diet restriction should always be combined with exercise in order to prevent an undesired loss of lean muscle tissue along with desired losses in excess or stored fat.

So take your time about weight loss, just as you pace yourself in other aspects of fashioning a permanent commitment to wellness-oriented living.

Spot Reduction: Forget it. Nature will not cooperate. The body system does not work this way. You cannot choose where excess fat will go when putting it on, nor do you have a vote on which sites it is taken off from. Why? Because fat loss is a condition of total calories expended, not *where* expended. Expect fat loss to occur first at the site of your most recent fat gains.

Put the large muscles of your legs to work first—you will burn more calories per unit of exercise time this way.

Spot exercise *will* burn some calories and *will* lead to better muscle tone in areas that sag from fat accumulation and muscle atrophy. But focus on whole-body endurance (aerobic) exercises that burn calories, strengthen the heart muscle, and diminish fat stores. In this fashion, your toning efforts will be genuine, not cosmetic.

Your Beliefs: Working For or Against Weight Loss

Whether you are chronically obese or just struggling with a few extra pounds, you will benefit from understanding how your beliefs contour your shape. Consider the following:

1. Describe what your life would be like if you woke up tomorrow morning and were miraculously at your ideal weight. Specifically, what would change?

   _____

   _____

   _____

2. What would remain the same as it is now if you were slender?

   _____

   _____

   _____

3. How will those closest to you react to your new figure?

   _____

   _____

   _____

4. What will you have to change in order to reach and maintain your ideal body weight?

   _____

   _____

   _____

5. Can you identify anyone whom you blame for being overweight? If so, who?

   _____

   _____

   _____

6. Why do you find it difficult to maintain a desirable weight?

_____

_____

_____

7. What excuses do you use to prevent yourself from being fit?

_____

_____

_____

8. How much longer do you plan to be out of shape?

_____

_____

_____

9. When do you plan on beginning your program?

_____

_____

_____

How about now? Only you can design a successful weight loss plan which takes into account your unique set of beliefs and behaviors. There is no ready-made approach. Remember, the major weight-control benefit of exercise does not come from the activity itself, whether it be jogging, hiking, swimming, or belly-dancing. Even strenuous activity _in itself_ does not use a vast amount of calories (a 20-minute run burns about 180—which you regain with a single glass of milk). The real benefit from exercise is changed muscle chemistry—for hours after exercise. Exercised muscles are better at sending out enzymes which pull fat from the bloodstream and use it for fuel—even as you rest. Exercised muscles become denser and leaner—they look better and so do you.

The Revolutionary ARDELL/TAGER PLAN For Weight Control

We realize that some people will want to ignore the realities, reject the long-term solutions, and continue the quest for the easy answer. Some of our methodical lifestyle suggestions may work for you, but we realize that this probably will not change the world. Too bad. If only there were a completely original solution, a scientific breakthrough, a revolutionary quick fix. Voilà! We have the perfect solution. Here is our fallback approach for people who are not yet ready for the slower Planning for Wellness method. We call this "The Vertical Hills Plan."

Think of it this way. No one is fat. Some are just *under height* for their weight. Our Vertical Hills Plan will make you taller! The plan requires no will power, no exercise, no real changes, and is instantaneous. Thus, we expect it will be a best seller, we will soon be on all the top TV shows, and we will be denounced by the AMA—which will make the Vertical Hills Plan even more popular.

Just consider this: No matter what you weigh, you are probably under weight for someone who is 6 feet, 5 inches. What's more, you are positively anorexic for one 6 feet, 11 inches. The problem, at the moment, is you are only 5 feet, 2 inches. That's why you need our Vertical Hills approach. In three months, you will grow at least six inches.

So remember, attitude is everything: you are not 65 pounds too much. You are one and a half feet too little. Get a grip on yourself. Forget horizontal—think vertical. Forget pounds—think inches.

We know our system works. We have used it with infants, tots, and adolescents. Using our Vertical Hills Plan, they have gained not just inches, but feet. (If you are already 6 feet or more, you may want to exercise caution in applying our methods. Too much success could be embarrassing and inconvenient, unless you like basketball.)

However, in the best of capitalist traditions, we will not reveal the secrets of the "Vertical Hills Plan." Until our next book. . . .

Formulating Your Plan

From the preceding pages you probably have an idea of where you need to place your emphasis if you are going to be successful in losing pounds and keeping them off. Here are two studies of the Planning for Wellness system in action against unwanted pounds. We hope you will be inspired by the creativity of these efforts.

Case 1—Roberta Dalton, a graduate student, decided that of the goals she selected, weight loss would be the most beneficial. Here's how she created her plan.

- The goals I set for myself are:
  1. I will improve my eating habits.
  2. I will lose six pounds by the end of the month.
  3. I will invite three friends to dinner each month.
  4. I will stop chewing gum.
- The payoffs I will receive are:
  1. I will become more alert and better able to study.
  2. I will fit into my summer wardrobe.
  3. I will have a better self image.
  4. I will realize that meal times can become special occasions to get together with my friends in a leisurely manner.
  5. I will save money by not purchasing junk food filled with empty calories.
- My goal-supporting activities are:
  1. I will eat a whole grain cereal breakfast every morning before leaving for school
  2. I will allow myself only dry popcorn for a snack after 7 p.m.
  3. I will eat fish or chicken three times a week.
  4. I will reduce my red meat consumption to less than one pound per week.
  5. I will eat one meal a day consisting of vegetable and whole grain combinations.
  6. I will drink only one cup of coffee a day.
  7. I will eat two fruits a day.
  8. I will weigh myself every third day and plot my progress.
- Friends who will assist me are:
  1. Tom, who works at the natural foods restaurant.
  2. Louise, whom I usually go drinking with, will remind me to stick to fruit juice.
  3. My mother will stop buttering my toast.
  4. My sister will keep fruit on the table.
- I know I have reached my goal when:
  1. I can concentrate more effectively.
  2. Tom and my sister notice my new figure.
  3. I don't crave junk food.
  4. I can get going in the morning without 3 cups of coffee.
- I realize I might sabotage my plan by:
  1. Not really changing any eating habits and just losing weight by starving myself or using diet pills.
- I will avoid this by:
  1. Sharing my record of when and what I eat with my class members and assessing the nutritional quality of my diet.

Case II—By his own admission, Glenn has been fat for four years. He finally decided to do something about it when one day while at the beach he realized he was beginning to look "like a beached whale."

Glenn decided it was time to take action. He developed a plan, and signed a contract with himself, witnessed by his wife, thereby enlisting her support and encouragement. Glenn then set out to carefully analyze his diet with the use of standard food composition charts—calculating the total number of calories and the number of grams of both fat and carbohydrates. He graphed these three measurements daily. Here's what his chart looked like at the ten-week point.

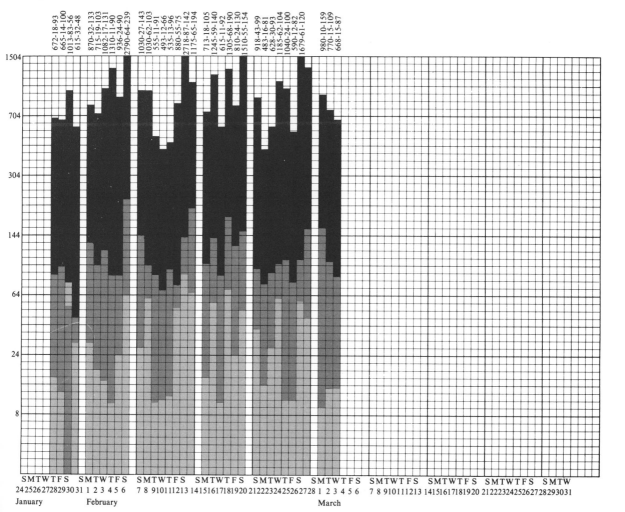

Carbohydrate (in grams)
Calories
Fat (in grams)

Glenn also charted his weight loss progress—and shared his record with a group of friends who were working on similar goals. The horizontal line represents his reward point—when he would share a delightful night on the town with his wife.

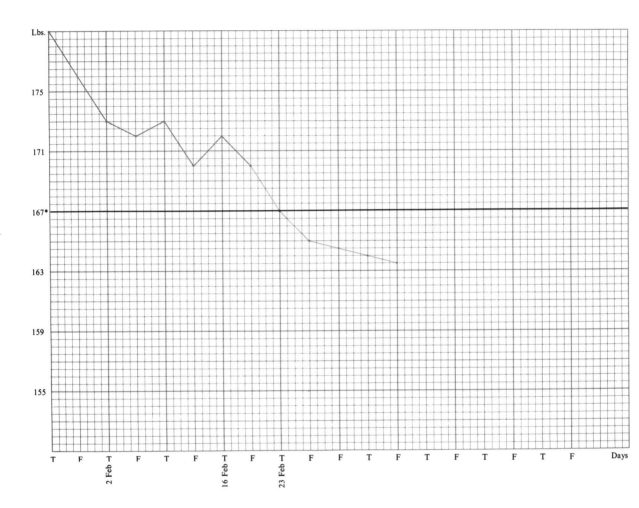

Charting weight loss progress is most valuable over long periods of time. Because weight may fluctuate widely from day to day, it is best to weigh yourself weekly. Be prepared to accept plateaus and minor setbacks. Remember your goal is long-term change.

An Evocative Exercise:
Stress Management

The word *stress* conjures up different images for people. To a physicist, stress might describe the shearing force applied to an object. To a psychologist, it might mean a response to a threat, whether real or imagined. To a laborer, it could be hauling a heavy weight up a hill, or having to endure excessive noise and dust. Stress is different things to different folks, but it is also some of the same things for many of us.

For most, for example, stress means tension. It means a vague uneasiness, an uptightness, a sense of pressure or urgency. It is often synonymous with frustration, an inability to accomplish a task, meet an expectation, or feel in control.

Stress accumulates when changes take place in our lives. It increases when we are unable to express feelings or to make needs and desires known. It compounds when our minds refuse to release persistent worries.

Yet stress is not all bad. It is, in fact, a basic force of life which can allow us to reach higher levels of performance. When managed properly, stress is a powerful ally for growth and accomplishment.

The "secret," of course, lies in an ability to manage tension levels. This begins with an ability to recognize the signs that it is *time* to manage stress.

If you purchase a new car, rototiller, chain saw, or other machinery, you will receive a maintenance manual. This will describe how to use and care for your new machine without stressing it beyond its capabilities. Humans do not come with such owner's instructions, perhaps because the gods believe that good care and thoughtful nurturance should be self-evident. We do not presume to be authorized to create a maintenance manual, but a few suggestions on stress awareness and management might be helpful. Later, you might even write your own manual for others.

A good place to start is in the area of recognizing warning signs of over-stress, and taking creative steps to get centered and balanced. In this way, we can live without allowing our biological equipment to suffer a breakdown as a result of poor response to stressful situations. It is important that we understand our own individual responses to pressure.

In general, we react in one of the three ways: with signs and symptoms, thoughts and feelings, or behaviors. Take a moment to look at the following figures. Circle those symptoms/feelings/behaviors which correspond to how you react.

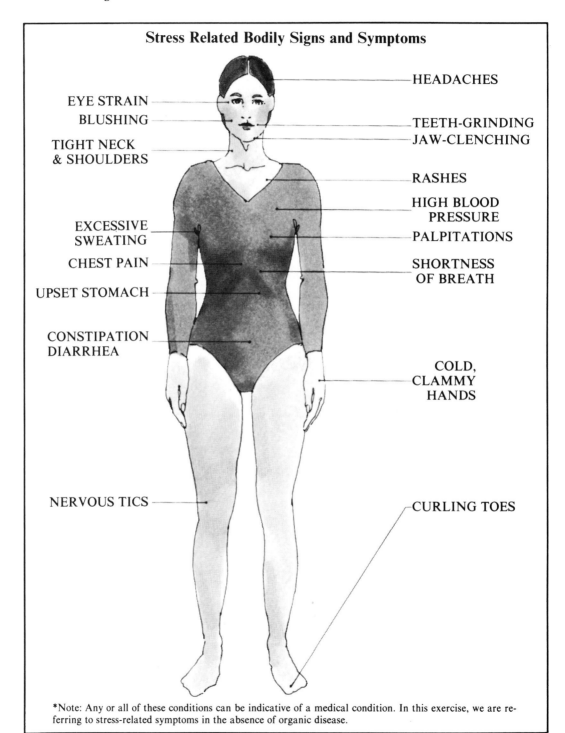

Stress Related Bodily Signs and Symptoms

HEADACHES

EYE STRAIN
BLUSHING

TEETH-GRINDING
JAW-CLENCHING

TIGHT NECK
& SHOULDERS

RASHES

HIGH BLOOD
PRESSURE

EXCESSIVE
SWEATING

PALPITATIONS

CHEST PAIN

SHORTNESS
OF BREATH

UPSET STOMACH

CONSTIPATION
DIARRHEA

COLD,
CLAMMY
HANDS

NERVOUS TICS

CURLING TOES

*Note: Any or all of these conditions can be indicative of a medical condition. In this exercise, we are referring to stress-related symptoms in the absence of organic disease.

Stress-related thoughts and feelings

- Depression
- Anger
- Forgetfulness
- Irritability
- Negative thoughts about oneself
- Apathy
- Altered sexual drive
- Impatience
- Bossiness

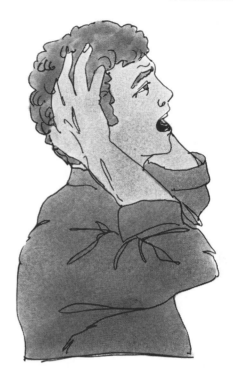

Stress-related behaviors:

- Increase or decrease in eating
- Increase in smoking
- Increase or decrease in sleeping
- Increase in drinking
- Reckless driving
- Compulsive gum chewing, whistling or laughing

Now take just a moment to recollect a recent stressful event which evoked these responses.

In a few short phrases, jot down what transpired and how you reacted.

Example: I was expected to meet three deadlines but had only enough time to complete one of them properly. I could feel my temples throbbing. I felt anxious and insecure, thought about quitting, and finally decided to do what I

could (knowing it would not be enough). _____

_____

_____

_____

Now ask yourself, Could you have responded in another way?

Yes _____   No _____

Was it inevitable that you would experience those feelings, thoughts or reactions?

Yes _____   No _____

Who was responsible for creating those signs or symptoms?

Me _____   Them _____

These three simple questions can get at the heart of your ability to handle stress. They acknowledge that although you often cannot control the events which create tension, you can control your response to them. No one else creates your headache, neck pain, or stomach acidity.

In psychological terms, allowing others to provoke these reactions in you means that you are giving your power to them. One way of retaining and strengthening your own personal power is to cultivate the appropriate attitude as a first line of defense.

Unless you plan to move to a mountain cave in the Himalayas and renounce your worldy cares and desires, chances are that the future has a storehouse of stressful events for you. Some of these you may already be anticipating (i.e., the inevitability of your 10-year-old becoming a teenager); others are beyond your wildest dreams . . . or nightmares. (In 1970, who ever envisioned that gasoline would be well over a dollar a gallon?)

To help you manage these "future trips," we have recently invented an amazing new device which can enable you to improve your attitude toward stress. Yes, dear reader, the "Retrospectoscope," not sold in any store, is our answer to stress management. When used according to directions, it promises to change your life. The Retrospectoscope, to exaggerate a bit, will enable you to sleep trouble-free, to run long distances effortlessly, to melt away tension and relax with ease, and to move ahead with balance and control of your life.

But first, before we put this marvelous instrument in your hands, let us give you a brief history of the origins of this unique wellness device.

Using the Retrospectoscope

Have you ever looked back on a stressful situation or event and wished you had said or done something differently? We would be surprised if not; most of us can think of circumstances where an instant replay would be desirable.

The passage of time often allows us to gain insight into past events. In heated conflicts, it is frequently difficult to be objective. Feelings of pride, envy, or anger obscure our judgment. When these feelings have had a chance to die down, we often have a clearer perspective.

What is not easy, of course, is maintaining this perspective during emotional states. If only we had a way to see clearly enough to either prevent or limit life's stresses and their effects upon us!

Enter the Retrospectoscope. This inexpensive tool, which you can construct at home, is the perfect way to help yourself remember. In order for the Retrospectoscope to be effective, however, it must be used according to the instructions below.

How to Construct Your
Retrospectoscope

1. Draw lines on a piece of 8½ × 11 paper as shown in the figure on the left.
2. With a scissors, cut out the shape you have drawn.
3. Roll and tape the paper so as to form a cone as in the figure on the right.
4. Now hold the large end up to your eye.
5. When you have seen enough, place the Retrospectoscope on your desk.
6. Feel free to color and decorate your retrospectoscope as desired. Some people prefer to write slogans on theirs, such as:
   "One Day At A Time."
   "It's Mighty Bad Now—Might Have Been Worse."
   "Never Play Leapfrog with a Unicorn."

Of course, unlike the other exercises, we do not expect you to do all the cutting and pasting to actually construct one of these ridiculous instruments. Visualizing the procedure should be sufficient.

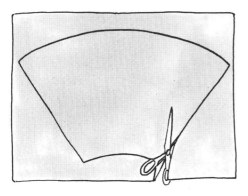 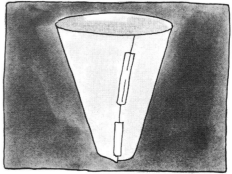

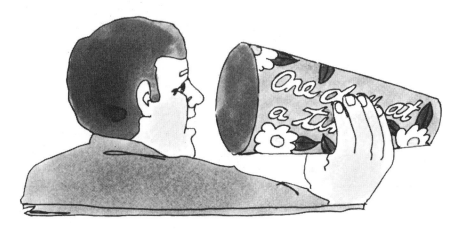

How to Use Your Retrospectoscope

The following conditions have been shown to enhance the effectiveness of your Retrospectoscope:

- laughter—directly proportional
- a healthy irreverence for ponderous business matters
- cultivating 5-year-olds as friends
- holding sand in your hands
- celebrating Halloween monthly
- other zany diversions

Interpretation

There is one problem with the Retrospectoscope. Most folks forget to use it soon enough. We've heard all sorts of excuses like, "Oh, I left it at the office" or "It's raining."

Pick it up right now. Close your eyes. Think of the last time you felt anger, embarrassment, anxiety, or fear. Now open your right eye and peer into the Retrospectoscope. Ask yourself what you can learn from that event, given the insights glimpsed with your marvelous new toy. Remember the Retrospectoscope is only a learning tool. When you use it, be gentle on yourself. It should not be used to browbeat yourself.

In addition to learning to use the Retrospectoscope there are a few additional skills which will help you manage stress.

Time Management

It's an all-too-common barrier—"no time." Yet we all have the same number of seconds, minutes and hours in the day. How is it, then, that some people accomplish so much, and others relatively little? The answer lies in effective time management.

Here are eight tips to help you plan better:

1. **Consolidate Similar Tasks.** For example, pay all household bills at one time, once or twice a month. Group outgoing phone calls together and make them all at one time—while you are set up with paper, pencil, and phone book.

2. **Tackle tough jobs first.** Start your day with the important work while your energy level is high, and work your way down your list of priorities. Leave busy-work chores until later in the day.

3. **Delegate responsibility.** Many "stress victims" think that the only way to get something done right is to "do it yourself". Training others and motivating them to do tasks you customarily perform can reduce time burdens in the future. This applies to friends as well as children and co-workers.

4. **Stem the paper tide.** Throw out junk mail (immediately), cancel unused subscriptions, re-route mail to others when appropriate. If possible, handle each piece of paper once, and don't pick up a piece of paper unless you plan to take some action.

5. **Avoid the cluttered-desk syndrome.** Clear your desk of everything except the work you intend to do during the day. Irrelevant work will remain out of sight, and out of mind.

6. **Chip away at important tasks.** Everyone faces unwelcome jobs from time to time. One good approach is to break the project down into "bite-size" pieces. Do a little every day. One advantage of this technique is that you get to stop sooner.

7. **Reduce meeting time.** Oh, how some meetings can d-r-a-g on. Try to schedule meetings that bump up against the lunch hour or quitting time, so all participants will be motivated to attend to business and leave. A more radical approach is the stand-up meeting, a technique which nearly always guarantees a short session.

8. **Take time to plan.** Paradoxically, taking time to plan can result in saving time in the long run. For example, a well-planned shopping expedition can save miles, hours, and dollars. Planning-oriented phone calls can cut down on time.

Breathe

Go ahead, in fact, and take a deep, relaxing breath. Perhaps you will notice a slight calming effect on your mind and your body. No doubt you can at least recall a situation when such a breath was associated with a feeling of relief, as in "whew!" We like to think of this kind of breathing as first aid—the immediate response, first learned but later automatic, to stressful situations.

You can use this technique anywhere. The kids just harvested your favorite houseplant: *breathe.* You are thirty miles from home, it's snowing, and the car won't start: *breathe.* You have just learned of a serious illness in the family, or fallen and broken an arm: again, long, slow breathing can help.

Simplistic? Deep breathing *is* simple, yes—but remembering to do it in crisis situations is not.

Cultivate Creative Outlets

Do something out of the ordinary. Play music, go to a play, attend the symphony, visit galleries, offer to give a speech on some arcane topic, or look into something that interests you but previously seemed too much trouble.

Stretch

Desk-bound mental activity creates tension in the neck and shoulders. The simple neck roll—moving the head around in a circle, slowly—can do much to alleviate tension and prevent it building up into pain. A shoulder shrug (bring the shoulders to the ears on inhalation, and completely and instantly drop them on exhalation) may also relieve muscle stress. The shoulders may be rotated in a circular motion also. Trading short neck rubs with a partner is also a good idea. A few toe-touches, some side-stretches and you will save yourself the stress that comes from chronic muscular tension.

Walk

Take short walks for no purpose other than to take short walks. Note the color of the air, the smell of the trees, the ambience of homes along your path. Plan no route, leave your wallet and watch at home, and above all, don't count your steps.

Ease Up on the Coffee

Sure the stuff wires you. How about switching to juices, herbal teas, and water? While you are at it, how about bringing some whole foods to work with you so you won't be tempted by the junk-food machines?

Learn a Relaxation Technique

The visualization described on page 26 is an excellent relaxation device. By practicing this exercise ten or fifteen minutes each day, you will learn to relax easily. The bibliography also contains several first-rate references on relaxation techniques.

Managing On-the-Job Stress

The Meaning of Work: A Wellness Perspective

For more than 100 million Americans, work consumes 37% of waking time. Often more when time spent thinking about it, and getting to and from it, is included. It's a major part of life, and has a big impact on our health.

Among other things, work contributes to our self-image. We label ourselves secretaries, doctors, lawyers, machinists, sanitation workers, and so on. And we develop personal identities consistent with work images.

All too often work becomes synonymous with stress. We equate our jobs with signs and symptoms of tension. We may well blame our ill feelings on co-workers, management, or that nebulous entity known as "the company." If we were into pointing fingers, it would be very expedient at this point to either (a) blame your job for your woes, or (b) criticize you for not actively managing your health to prevent work-related burn-out. Though tempting, this would be both inaccurate and futile.

Work stress is really a shared proposition. Managing it requires developing the attitudes and skills which will enable you to cope with the inevitable hassles of working life. In addition, it requires that your company moderate physical and other work stresses to a manageable level.

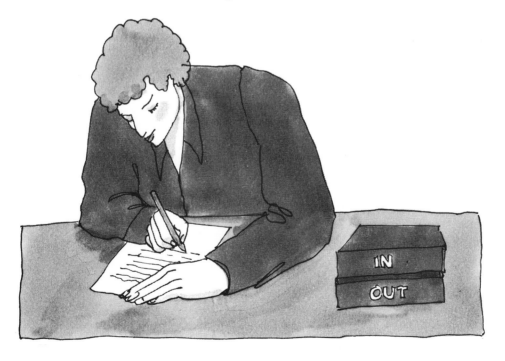

You will find a comprehensive outline of how to go about changing your company's environment to include a wellness program in chapter five of PLANNING FOR WELLNESS. Right now let's focus on some of the personal questions which you'll need to answer in order to manage self-imposed work stressors. We'll begin by helping you understand what you want from your job. Take a few minutes and complete the open-ended phrases listed below. Respond quickly with the first answer that comes to mind. This questionnaire can also form the basis for an informative group discussion with your co-workers.

The Meaning of Work Exercise

1. In general, I feel that work is _____

_____

_____

2. What I would like from my job is _____

_____

_____

_____

3. The greatest frustration in my work is _____

_____

_____

4. The greatest joy in my work is _____

_____

_____

5. The demands of my job _____

_____

_____

6. I realize that my present work cannot fulfill the following needs _____

_____

_____

7. I am able to get these needs met by _____

_____

_____

8. I would consider leaving my job _____

_____

_____

Interpretation

Before you can begin to plan for improved job satisfaction, you must understand how you feel about work in general and your job in particular. Not everyone can change jobs easily. So it's important to begin to identify your work-related needs. The questions listed above help you do that. If you have been tempted to skip over them to get to the next section, we urge you to reconsider. Go back and fill them out now.

To further clarify your own philosophy and beliefs about work, please examine the phrases listed below. Place an X on the line closest to the statement with which you agree.

For me, work is a means to an end.		Work is a growth opportunity.
−10	0	+10
I put in my time to make money.		In my work, I have exciting challenges which test my abilities.
−10	0	+10

I derive all my satisfactions and joys in life from other activities besides work.		I can find a lot of satisfaction in being creative and innovative at work.
−10	0	+10
At the end of the day, I can easily put my job aside and do other things which are important to me.		At the end of the day, I still think about my job even when at home or during play.
−10	0	+10
I believe that work is something I have to do to get by.		I believe that work itself is and should be enriching and satisfying.
−10	0	+10

People are drawn to their professions for a variety of reasons. Obviously your work philosophy and your training helped shape your selection of a particular job. But jobs themselves have specific attributes which make them unique. They differ in physical characteristics (such as time spent sitting, lifting, stooping, standing), level of responsibility, time requirements and financial remuneration.

A preponderance of marks on the right-hand side indicates a greater level of involvement with your work. It means that your expectations and job stresses are potentially greater, but so are your rewards. If you find yourself far to the left side in all or most of the areas noted, you might want to creatively consider ways to derive greater satisfaction from your daily routine.

An essential question which you need to ask yourself about your present job is whether the characteristics of the job are compatible with your underlying work philosophy. If not, your performance will suffer.

Expectations and Actualities: Two Cases

Sandra Livingwell is a college graduate who majored in business economics before coming to work as assistant personnel manager for Telex Communications, Ltd. In accepting the position, Sandra looked forward to working with troubled employees, assisting them with their problems. She was also drawn to Telex by perceived opportunities for rapid advancement and increasing job responsibility. A dedicated problem-solver, Sandra is an avid chess player who travels to compete in several major tournaments each year.

In the last two years, eighty percent of Sandra's working time has been devoted to compiling the company's disability statistics. Sandra finds the work tedious and unimaginative. She reports to work at 8:00 and leaves promptly at 5:00.

Despite repeated inquiries, her boss seems unwilling to increase the scope of her job to include more personal interactions. He is also reluctant to provide her with greater decision-making capability. Frustrated and bored, Sandra is resigned to stick it out until she can find more challenging work within the company or elsewhere.

Charlie Turbo has worked as a machinist at Telex Communications, Ltd., for over 12 years. He remembers when the company was first started. There were only three machinists then; now there are over 300. Charlie is a good machinist. Stamping out the mechanical parts one after another has a special rhythm for him. He leaves work with a sense of accomplishment at the end of a productive day. Other than the infrequent days when he has disagreements with his supervisor—usually over a technical point—he rarely leaves work thinking about his job.

Charlie enjoys the camaraderie in the machine shop. After work he frequently stops for a beer with several of his longtime co-workers.

Things changed when Charlie was promoted to shop foreman. Suddenly it seemed the problems were never-ending—forms to fill out, government regulations with which to comply, committees to coordinate, and personnel problems to sort out. At first elated by the increased salary and prestige, Charlie's wife became less enthusiastic as her husband became increasingly inattentive, tired, and irritable. Further, Charlie's ulcer flared up and that did not make him any more agreeable.

Interpretation

In the cases sketched above, there is an obvious imbalance between job expectations and actualities. Both workers experience stress overloads as a result of the way they choose to react to their job conditions.

Sandra and Charlie are most comfortable with opposite extremes on the spectrum listed on the following page.

Sandra's Job Attributes and Expectations	Charlie's Job Attributes and Expectations
Variable routine	Predictable routine
Decision-making ability	Following orders
Freedom to make choices	Clear-cut job definition
Initiate organizational changes	Follow organizational changes
Self-starter	Closely supervised

Obviously, Sandra and Charlie are matched with jobs that provide a poor fit, given their values and preferences. Too bad they cannot switch places; Sandra would probably be a superb machine shop foreman.

Job satisfaction is dependent on a number of interrelated factors. First and foremost, it helps a great deal if you are convinced of the importance of the job to be done. As we saw in the two case studies, the job must blend with underlying personal values.

No matter how rigidly structured your job may be, it is important for you to recognize that everyone can make important changes in his or her job. There is a front- and a back-door way. We recommend, except as a last resort, a polite knock on the front door.

The Job Change Exercise

Take a stab at discovering what you can change by completing the following sentence. The aspects of my job which I would *like* to change are _____

_____

_____

_____

_____

Now, try this: If I were a clever devil, I probably *could* change _____

_____

_____

_____

_____

Stumped? Can't think of a thing? Perhaps if you could overhear a short subway conversation between the old work ethic and the creative work ethic, some ideas might come to mind.

Old Work Ethic: "Times are tough. You gotta keep your nose to the grindstone, kiddo, and don't rock the boat . . . Besides, you can't change your job, anyway."

Creative Work Ethic: "Sure, I know there are some things that I'll never be able to change about my job. However, while I cannot expect to achieve 100% of what I want, there are important things I can do."

Old Work Ethic: "Oh yeah, like what?"

Creative Work Ethic: "Like working to change the balance within my job. I can get a sense of newness and variety by juggling my writing, phoning, sitting, meeting, planning, and daydreaming time."

Old Work Ethic: "Well, that's easy to do if you are a manager, but what about us production workers?"

Creative Work Ethic: "There is no standard way, but everyone can change something. On an assembly line, you can change your involvement with others and the physical work environment. Consider a number of mental games, banter, group contests, musical accompaniment, potluck parties, and fitness activities for starters."

Assume for a moment you could do just about anything to make the job or your time on the job more interesting. Do not censor yourself. Make a list of what you could do.

1. _____
2. _____
3. _____
4. _____
5. _____
6. _____

Finished? Go back and place a check next to those that might, with a little planning, be feasible.

Have others at the workplace make a similar list—just for fun. Compare notes. Finally, see if you have come up with some practical ideas.

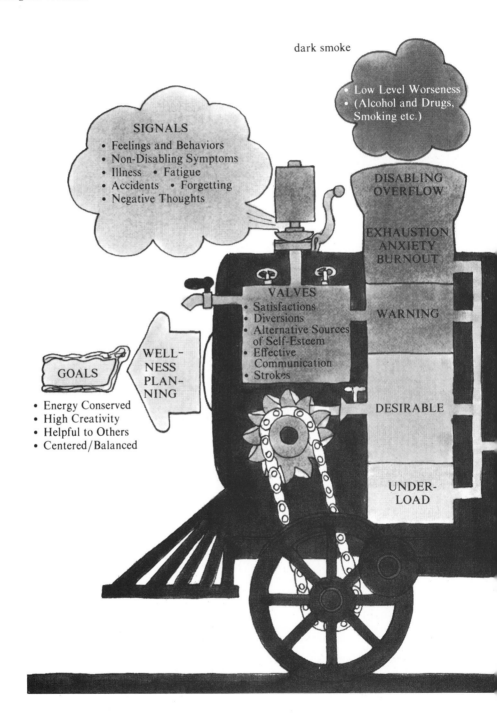

dark smoke

SIGNALS
- Feelings and Behaviors
- Non-Disabling Symptoms
- Illness • Fatigue
- Accidents • Forgetting
- Negative Thoughts

- Low Level Worseness
- (Alcohol and Drugs, Smoking etc.)

DISABLING OVERFLOW

EXHAUSTION ANXIETY BURNOUT

WARNING

VALVES
- Satisfactions
- Diversions
- Alternative Sources of Self-Esteem
- Effective Communication
- Strokes

DESIRABLE

WELL-NESS PLAN-NING

GOALS
- Energy Conserved
- High Creativity
- Helpful to Others
- Centered/Balanced

UNDER-LOAD

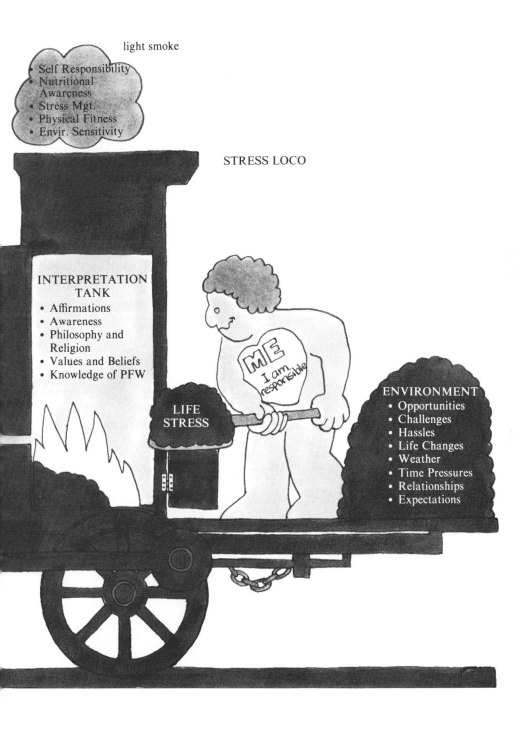

Try it. It may not work out, but you can't be sure until you have made an effort. Even the process will help.

Managing on-the-job stress requires that we understand what it is we want from our work, how we can redesign our job for enhanced satisfaction, and how we can join together with management and co-workers (See p. 135) to develop supportive health environments.

Managing stress is a continual balancing act. By attempting to meet our goals, take on new responsibilities, and learn new skills, attitudes and behaviors, we choose to use the energy of stress, rather than have it use us. We also must learn to react to the inevitable external environmental stressors without being knocked off track. Here's where the retrospectoscope can help us interpret events as opportunities—not crises.

There is an optimum level of tension which we require in order to perform well. When stress exceeds that level, exhaustion and burnout are the result. Each of us must become aware of the signals from the body when our stress has exceeded the safe zone, and plan appropriate ways to reduce the disabling overflow.

Finally, and most critically, we must cultivate positive means of dealing with tension. We can achieve satisfaction from successfully channeling stress energies toward positive outcomes. As shown on the "stress locomotive," a knowledge of the dynamics of stress (fuel) fires our bodies (locomotive) for better (light smoke) or worse (dark smoke). When the mix isn't right, speed and efficiency are lost (listen for the whistle). When stress is managed and well-channelled (right mixture), the train roars down the track—and life goals are reached.

Now you have all the theory you need—including everything you ever wanted to know about the wellness concept, the personal wellness planning process, and wellness skills. What could be left? . . . save to apply all this good theory to making wellness a reality at home, work, and play.

Chapter
4

Wellness at Home

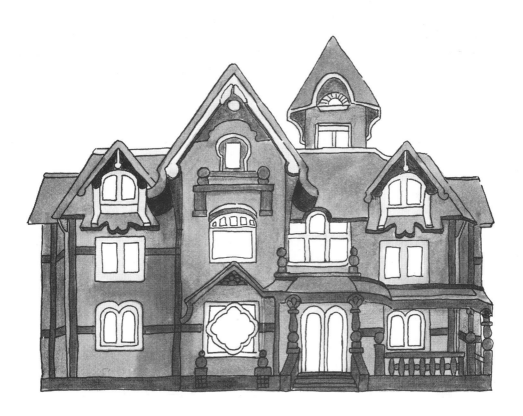

Let's proceed now to look at the potential impact of Planning for Wellness system on the home. The exercises in this chapter are designed to help you build skills in applying wellness principles at home.

Is there a place for wellness concepts in your home, an openness to integrating wellness principles into your home life? According to one recent survey entitled "Family Health in an Era of Stress"* (by Yankelovich, Skelly, and White) conducted for General Mills, there surely seems to be growing interest in health throughout the U.S. "The majority of American families are ready to accept in principle a new and more active approach to health and health care . . . aimed primarily at preventing health problems before they arise."

Of course, an openness to acceptance and an impressive track record are not the same thing. The report continues: "yet only a minority are beginning to put these new beliefs into action . . . [by making] the lifestyle changes necesary to improve their health."

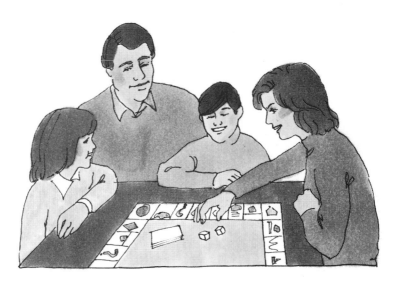

As mentioned in our first chapter, wellness planning allows participants to narrow the gap between intention and action. The home provides numerous opportunities for family members to shape a wellness lifestyle.

What does the home represent? Among other things we could label the home as:

*"Family Health in an Era of Stress," is available from General Mills, Inc., P.O. Box 1113, Minneapolis, Minnesota 55440.

- **The main computer** where family members store the shared beliefs and values which reinforce their sense of connectedness to each other and to the world around them. The bonding between family members serves as the nucleus for the skills of socializing.

  The association between the quality of family ties and optimal health is supported by more than common sense. Plentiful data from epidemiological research underscores the strength of this association. In a nine-year study of mortality in 4,725 adults between the ages of 30 and 69 years in Alameda County, researchers Berkman and Syme,* investigated the effects of four types of social contact upon longevity. These four types of contact included marriage, frequency of visits with friends and relatives, church attendance, and participation in formal and informal groups. The study showed that the risk of death was 2.8 times higher in the women and 2.3 times higher in the men with the fewest, as compared with the most, social ties.

- **A script-writing center** for the evolution of self-concept in childhood and early adolescence. It provides powerful role remodeling during the years when a young person is trained, directly and by example, to want to assume responsibility and pursue excellence. The young child's early associations with Mr. Yuk, seat belts and fire prevention provide the spring board for self-responsibility in the years ahead.

  The home influence is equally important as the child reaches his teens. The preteen and teenage years are times of physical change, social anxiety, and uncertain purposes. This is even truer today, with our drugs, expanding sexual options, new technology, economy, and the Bomb. The consequences: 34 percent of our young have risk factors for coronary heart disease before the age of 20, roughly half of American youth experiment with illicit drugs, alcohol and unprotected premarital intercourse. This year 600,000 women under the age of 19 will become pregnant. Venereal disease has increased 200% among 15- to 19-year olds, and 163 percent among 10- to 14-year-olds.

  Most teenagers still find it difficult to discuss health subjects with their parents, although, according to Yankelovitch, they welcome open and frank discussion about sex. Yet studies indicate that parents are potentially the most effective sex educators for their children, and help prevent teenage pregnancy. Of course, this requires not only the learning of communication skills, but the development of relationships which foster respect, trust and acceptance.

---

*L. F. Berkman, and S. L. Syme, "Social Networks, Host Resistance, and Mortality: A Nine-Year Followup of Alameda Residents," *AMJ Epidemiology Log:* 186–204, 1979.

- **A transition center,** a "Grand Central Station" from where children, parents, and grandparents make connections to all the major points and places in life (e.g., schools, jobs, and so on). As a station, the home is where you must learn how to read schedules (know the rules), ask directions (learn from those older and wiser), manage vendors (balance demands), and enjoy the time at hand (have fun).

  The American family itself is in transition. Roles are being challenged, tested, and redefined. Look at women, for example. Who would have imagined, say in 1940, that working wives would outnumber housewives in the 1980's, or that 42 percent of working women would be the sole support of their families? Finally, there are older people. We live longer than in 1940 or any other time for that matter, but are we living better? The current number is 25 million aged 65 and over in North America.* By the year 2000, it will be nearly double this figure, barring nuclear and other disasters.

- **The training ground** for all required and extra-credit life skills, such as language, nutritional awareness, medical self-care and fitness enjoyment, to note just a few.

  The Yankelovitch study identified a lack of knowledge of basic health practices as a major obstacle preventing families from reaching higher levels of health. Another was confusion about the proliferation of government health warnings, which we believe turns people off when not marked by positive messages about the satisfactions possible with behavior changes.

  Fortunately, there are signs of encouragement. The number of joggers is unprecedented, health books are best sellers, the wellness movement is in full swing, and families are the focus in much of the institutional wellness programming. In this section, exercises are provided which you can use not only to learn about wellness for families, but have fun in the process.

- **A sacred place,** a temple or church of the soul and spirit. Regardless of creed dogma, tradition, or allegiance, it is the home environment which draws and inspires its residents to reflect on inner matters.

---

*Of course, if we have our way, there will be a new method of counting. In the wellness "new math," 65 will be considered middle age. Where do we put old age, assuming a wellness lifestyle? We cannot agree between us: Mark insists on 110; being a bit older, Don opts for 117.5. Time will tell or, as Parkinson has noted: "The future lies ahead."

Toward Healthy Relationships

Bookstores in recent years have found a rich market for self-help titles which urge us to look out for No. 1, pull our own strings and generally make our way through the world by manipulating it to our own advantage.

These books reaffirm an elemental truth—after all, if we don't look out for ourselves, who will?—but they also suggest a rather narrow psychology of life. Does psychological health really boil down to one dimensional self-interest?

Absolutely not. What happens when No. 1 realizes his main interest in life is suddenly a No. 2? Or when a No. 1, Jr. , arrives all wet and wiggly into this world? Psychologically, there is still a self-interest angle, but there is also something else: Love.

There are a few things in this life more important than personal comfort, more important even than health: Love is one of them. Paradoxically, the ability to allow our interest and concern to spread beyond the boundaries of our skin is one of the sure signs of mental well-being. To be totally self-possessed, self-absorbed, and self-serving is to run the risk of becoming totally sour. Mentally, it simply isn't healthy to get stuck on yourself. In fact, we can even say that the amount of real love in your life—the amount of caring, positive feelings for others—is an important index of your overall health and well-being. Thus, love is a wellness tool and an important one.

The late Erich Fromm, a popular psychologist-author of another era, reminded us loving is an art. In other words, love doesn't just happen. Some positive feelings for others do come naturally, but to thrive and endure, genuine love must be created. For most people, creative loving begins with one primary relationship. The art of sustaining a loving relationship with a main or number one friend is demanding, requires effort and, some say, luck. But success is possible, and the rewards are worth it.

Relationships are only as alive as the people engaging in them. As with every dimension of health, relationships also require monitoring, assessing, enhancing, and changing.

Let's now take a look at the most important qualities of relationships and determine whether your relationships are meeting your wellness requirements.

Get In Touch with Your Own Needs, Desires, and Expectations

Falling in love is wonderful . . . too bad its half-life is so short. Eventually, the magic of first romance fades and, to be successful, the relationship must match up to a more fundamental set of criteria. For a starter, complete the sentences below.

What I want in a relationship with ___(Name of Person)___ is . . . (list 10 minimum).

1.   6.

2.   7.

3.   8.

4.   9.

5.   10.

It's also important to know what draws you away from your partner. For example:

What I'm afraid of in my relationship with (Name of Person) is . . . (list 10 minimum)

1.   6.

2.   7.

3.   8.

4.   9.

5.   10.

On the answers listed above, place a star next to the two most meaningful issues for you. Now ask yourself, "Have I shared these thoughts and feelings with my partner?" If not, what's holding you back?

The answer may involve many things—fear of anger, disappointment or disillusionment. We often assume that others can read our minds and know our desires. Perhaps your needs may be inordinate or so fundamentally different that your partner can never fulfill them. Invariably, however, the long-term stress of not communicating these inner feelings is greater than whatever repercussions can arise from open dialogue.

Change the Type and Quality of Communication

- When you have a beef (or vegetable) with your partner, begin by expressing your feelings. Many of us have been brought up without knowing how to, or being given permission to, express our feelings. It *is healthy to express feelings, even (or especially) angry or upsetting emotions. An ability to pinpoint your emotions and express them in the first person (i.e., "I feel _____ .") can often short-circuit explosive arguments marked by hostility, blame, overkill, and guilt. Besides, who can argue about the way you feel?* Here are some helpful adjectives to be familiar with:

I feel _____

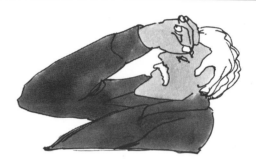

(pick one)

angry	let down
concerned	betrayed
perplexed	devalued
disappointed	used
confused	manipulated

(After reading this list, a long sigh and thirty seconds of tranquility are in order.)

- State your point of view. To communicate means more than just talking with another person. Express your side of a situation. Refrain from the need to prove the other person wrong. Try to be concise.
- Make certain the other person got your intended message. There are many reasons why people often do not get our messages. We may not have been clear in our presentation. We may have picked an inopportune moment to present our complaint, or the other person may have simply tuned out. People's attitudes, needs, values, present health status, or temperament can prevent them from hearing what you have to say. Encourage them to paraphrase what you've said. (You might also try asking your partner if it is O.K. to address a certain area before doing so. This can increase his or her receptivity to what you have to say.)
- Be willing to negotiate and accept a compromise. To negotiate means you, too, must be a good listener. You cannot always have everything your way, so some compromise is essential. Even in the best of situations good communication skills involve hearing the other person's point of view. Try not to interrupt.
- If appropriate, make an agreement to jointly act upon the problem. If you feel some change is in order and mutually agreed upon, write the steps you will be taking to implement the solution, make a firm but clear agreement, and consent to examine progress after a stipulated length of time.

- Remember that "strokes" are essential to good relationships. A stroke is a unit of recognition; it is a word, phrase, or gesture which acknowledges that you value your partner. Get in the habit not only of bestowing them on those around you, but on yourself as well. Feel free to ask for a stroke when you need it.
- These communication skills are valuable in a host of situations. They can be applied just as well in dealing with friends, coworkers, and others.

Spend More Quality Time Together

Quality time (QT) is a precious commodity. It is to relationships what clean air is to the environment—that is, integral.

It is not really true that familiarity breeds contempt; it merely begets forgetfulness of the importance of QT. We are confident that at some point in your life, you have enjoyed quality time with somebody. There is no need to dwell on what QT is, except to note that it includes a sense of being in the moment, free from the preoccupations of future expectations, plans and dreams, and past regrets, accomplishments, and delights. We think that QT is evident in relationships marked by:

- shared recreational activities
- holding hands
- writing and receiving a love letter*
- giving and receiving a message
- meditating together before or after making love
- sharing a meal in joy and appreciation
- reading a meaningful statement aloud
- music, art, dance

These are a few of our thoughts. How might you put some more QT into your relationships? What examples occur to you?

_____

_____

_____

_____

_____

*When was the last time you wrote or received one?

Define Role Expectations and Orientation

Managing a relationship is like running a business. Someone must be in charge of ordering the supplies, keeping the books, tightening up the shop and making sure quality products (e.g., kids) and services (e.g., personal growth) are created. This requires not only give and take, but clear delineation of responsibilities and expectations so that things run smoothly. In our culture today roles are shifting. Keeping abreast of your partner's expectations, let alone your own, requires constant vigilance.

For some couples, two very special areas of concern are handling of finances and raising children. In each case developing an understanding of your partner's expectations is critical for a harmonious relationship.

Work at Getting a Clearer Vision of How You Would Like Your Relationship To Be in the Future

We move toward, and become like, that which we think about.

A common vision can sustain a relationship through tough times by providing the larger perspective of long-term goals. A helpful means of establishing this vision is through the practice of mutual goal-setting. Here is how it works.

On a large piece of paper, write what you would both like your lives to be like in ten years. Note ideal future projections in such areas as economics, social status, general lifestyle, work situation, time allocation, living arrangements, traits you expect to develop in the next ten years, hobbies you would like to develop, professions you would like to pursue, possessions you would like to acquire. Feel free to portray some of these visually. Don't dwell on this; brainstorm your desired situations in less than five minutes. You need not exhibit any restraint—after all, anything and everything may be possible. Furthermore, what is not possible may be fun to think about.

When you have both completed your visions, examine them side by side. Look at the areas of overlap and the areas where you are poles apart. This can provide content for a valuable heart-to-heart discussion, including the following issues:

- What are your areas of common interest?
- How can these be highlighted and worked toward in practical ways?
- Under what conditions would you consider ending or changing the nature of your relationship?
- How willing are you to support your friend in those areas which are clearly related to his or her growth and really do not interest you that much?

All this is risky, of course, but risks are a part of growth and thus basic to QT.

• Recognize that relationships change. Relationships have their own natural cycles or phases. Initiating a relationship involves building upon common interests, learning from each other, and sharing experiences. Maintenance revolves more around protecting valued qualities and creatively keeping interest levels high. In includes a high level of acceptance and resisting the temptation to try to become, or make someone become, something he/she is not.

There is also an appropriate time to let go of a relationship. There is no one else who can tell you when your relationship has reached this point. If you find yourself in this position, review the content areas we have just covered. Determine whether your innermost needs are going unmet, despite ample communication. Examine your activities and ascertain whether you still derive enthusiasm from doing things together. Is the relationship nurturing your personal growth or merely presenting another set of obstacles? How about the deeper values of trust, respect and honesty? Have you kept these values intact, or are they irreparably damaged?

These are just a few of the soul-searching questions involved in dissolving a primary relationship. Letting go is a natural phase. Still, it isn't easy. Perhaps the best description of the dilemma is offered by Hillel in an often-quoted remark: "If I am not for myself, who will be? If I am only for myself, then what am I? And if not now, when?"

Wellness for Kids

Among the most potentially rewarding relationships are those which we have with our children. They offer stodgy old adults the priceless opportunity to become young again, to see the world through a fresher set of eyes.

Children are also one of life's greatest stressors. Our expectations for them are usually innumerable, but our patience is finite. As parents we expect straight "A's," clean rooms, perfect manners, and total obedience.

It's bad enough dealing with our expectations of our children. But we have them of ourselves as well. After all, who wouldn't like to be the perfect parent? (This is an even greater stressor for the single parent.) We all know that raising children is a full-time job, even though few of us have full time to do it. Like all jobs, some of us do better at it than others. But there is more to it than just being naturally cut out for the job; a good deal of training goes into successful parenting.

In recent years, a number of excellent books have been written about the art of parenting. All that we have read share a number of common principles which support the wellness philosophy. Among them are the following:

1. **There's enough punishment in life.** Yelling, screaming, scolding, beating—these are ineffective ways to get your message across to a child.

2. **Reward your child for positive behaviors.** The best way to encourage the development of good habits and attitudes is to reward a child when he or she displays them. Some of the best rewards are those which are social in nature. These include spending more time together, reading, allowing greater access to TV, staying up late, or engaging in a favorite hobby.

3. **Use effective punishers appropriately.** Kids like to be where the action is. One of the most effective means of getting your message across is by calling for time out; simply put the child off by him or herself for a few minutes in a room, a corner, or a quiet space until he or she calms down. Call it a penalty box, not a relaxation break, or else the kid will grow up hating the idea of stress management.

4. **Kids watch what you do.** Remember your actions speak louder than your words in raising children. It's important to be a good role model.

5. **Spend more time playing together.** After all, this is what kids do best. It's often their only chance to be experts. Learn to make creative use of the time you have together by structuring whole family wellness activities.

   We thought you might like a "for instance" or two, so we asked some friends what they do. The responses suggest that while there is no "right way" that would work for everybody, most can benefit and have fun by adapting certain principles. Take the Willard case, for example:

   The Willard Family identified "the problem." The breakfast table was always covered with jelly, crayons turned up in the strangest of places, toys and clothes were strewn about the house. The common spaces—kitchen, bathroom and living room—were perpetual disaster areas.

   Steve, age 34, and Karen, age 31, tried most of the familiar measures. They yelled, scolded, threatened and cajoled. Toys did get picked up, chores done, but sooner or later Chandy (age 8) and Carl (age 5) would lapse back into their familiar patterns. Even little Jesse (age 2) would get into the act. The situation improved vastly after the Willards developed their family wellness plan. The process was not only easy, but fun as well. Here's how it worked.

• During the weekly family meeting each child too young for goal statements would draw a picture of the chore/s they would be performing that week. The picture would be placed in a conspicuous location in the house (i.e., refrigerator, above calendar, next to phone).

- Carl and Chandy each made a list of favorite payoffs on 3 × 5 reward cards. These included:

  having a friend sleep overnight
  going roller skating
  taking the whole family to the movie of *their* choice
  play-wrestling with daddy ("You know, daddy is the horse and we all get to jump on him," said Carl.)
  having a picnic
  eating dinner out
  going to the zoo

  The cards were kept in a special reward box.
- Next, Karen obtained some fifty different stickers—wellness rainbows, happy face stars, unicorns, teddy bears, magic moons—which she would affix next to the children's drawings when they had completed their activity. Once a predetermined number of stickers was reached, Carl or Chandy would get their reward.

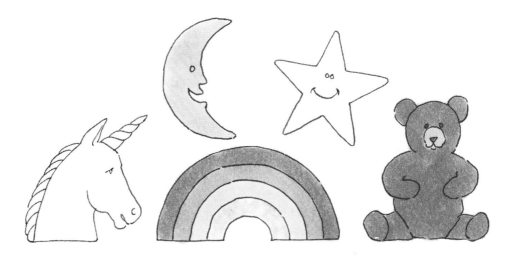

Sounds pretty simple—but plans such as these tell us a lot about wellness. In this case, the Willards not only taught self-responsibility, but got a cleaner house and, most important, reinforced the notion that the best rewards are the quality moments a family spends together.

Nutritional Awareness at Home

There is something special about sitting down for a meal with family members and other people who are special to you. It can be an occasion for celebration in a quiet and serene way; it can be a time for acknowledgment of someone's accomplishments; it can be a period to express commitments to oneself or others in an atmosphere of loving support and affection. It can be a time for all these things, and for limitless other ceremonies and rituals that bring people who are special even closer to each other—and to themselves. In an understated, low-key manner, every meal can have elements that create these effects.

Here is a simple activity which you can undertake at home with your parents, children, or close friends to encourage raised food awareness and a calm atmosphere at mealtime.

An Atmosphere Exercise for Mood Food

Make a list of everything that comes to your mind in three minutes (start timing *after* you have read the instructions and are ready to begin) that would add a quality of reflection, acknowledgment, calm, mutual support, or which would, in any desirable way, make every meal a special event.

There is only one rule for this exercise: Do not censor anything that comes to mind; be uninhibited. The ideas you list are not for every meal; variety is a spice that goes with dining as well as on the food.

Ready? Check your watch and go. _____

_____

_____

_____

_____

_____

_____

_____

Now, take a look at your list. Chances are that only a few of them look feasible. But the exercise is beneficial in that that you have had a bit of practice thinking of rituals and techniques for making the food experience at home somewhat distinguished. Now you are ready for the next step.

Announce to your family (or with whomever you share a home environment) that you have a new game to play. Give the game a jazzy title. Maybe "Food for *all* of you—not just your face" or something like that (you know what will sell in your household). Explain that the idea is to have fun in generating ideas for a real problem.

The problem, you can explain, is that it is hazardous to good digestion to eat quickly, disruptive of emotional well-being to be distressed/upset/out of sorts while dining, and unmindful of the opportunities for family harmony to overlook ceremony/tradition/reflection when everyone is together for meals. Therefore, you have a game that might lead to some new and beneficial practices.

Note that the only rule of the game is that there be no censoring. Everyone should write down, without discussing with others, whatever ideas occur to him or her. Give everybody three minutes.

When the time is up, have each person discuss his/her ideas. Again, it is best not to judge or debate the ideas, just hear everybody out. Next, everybody talks about what the experience of playing this game was like. Did you learn something? Are any of the ideas feasible? Is it a good idea to make something special of the meal hours?

Here is a list of some of the ideas we have heard in playing this game in our homes:

- Hold hands in silence for ten seconds and take three deep breaths.
- Hold hands and smile at each other (time required: three seconds).
- Take turns each day giving brief speeches on how great you were (or will be) today.
- Pretend that there is at the table, as guest, a world leader. One person acts out the role of the leader in addressing the rest of the family. Be brief.
- Read a favorite poem or passage from a book. Take turns doing this, or assign the task for an entire week to a volunteer.
- Discuss the nutrients in the foods to be eaten, the calories in each serving, and the role of the major vitamins and minerals found in each food in helping the body function at its best levels.
- Have each person estimate the percentage of the meal consisting of proteins, fats, and carbohydrates. (The cook, with a little research, should be able to come pretty close to judging these percentages.)
- Listen to reports on the progress each person might be making in carrying out his/her personal wellness plan.

- Thank the farmers, animals, and plants which have contributed in their own ways to make this meal possible.
- Acknowledge in some way your good fortune in living at a time and place where abundance as represented by this meal is possible.

Of course, there is only so much you can do with the mood or atmosphere aspect. Eventually you have to address the food issue itself. But these ideas should provide you with some thoughts on how you can make mealtime an enriching experience.

Wellness for Teens

The Mirage of Youth as a Freeway to Ruin

It is not so difficult to convince middle-aged folks that personal behaviors, attitudes, and what we call "lifestyle factors" make a big difference in their health status. They know people who have developed degenerative diseases. They have had friends die prematurely because of heart disease, cancer, stroke, and accidents. Even if their habits are less than ideal, they *do* understand the link between their health practices and their level of well-being.

Not so with a lot of teenagers. Many young people are "burdened" with myths and dysfunctional expectations which provide few exits off "the Freeway to Ruin."

What are the sights along this pernicious road? Here is a sampling of "billboard" advertisements found on this hazardous path:

- I can eat all the junk food I want because I don't have a weight problem.
- I can smoke if I want to. Kids don't get lung cancer. I'll stop when I am 30 or so.
- Why make a big deal out of health? Unless you really freak out, your body can take it.
- If only I looked like (person of your choice), then I'd have it made.
- I don't wear seatbelts because if I'm in a wreck, I'll be trapped.

Because of mass media stereotypes, peer pressure, and the absence of advertising for an attractive alternative like wellness, many young people believe these and similar myths. Unfortunately, this "mirage of youth" phenomenon prevents many adolescents from getting involved in health activities. Think just a moment about your health resources. Are you withdrawing more than you are depositing? As a teenager, you can get away with it—for a while—but these habits may make you a bad credit risk in the years ahead.

The exercises in *Planning For Wellness* can facilitate a reassessment of mirage-like beliefs. You can reevaluate some key beliefs in order to cope more realistically. These efforts will help you to become more open to life-enhancing values and behaviors. What is more important, you will be more attuned to constructive approaches to popularity and self acceptance, and less hooked on the need to go along with the crowd, sometimes at fearful costs to yourself and others.

The Jennie Smith Tragedy

One alternative course to the "freeway to ruin" is frank, open communication between adolescents and those whom they come in contact with on a regular basis (family, friends, and teachers). We offer the next exercise as a way to facilitate this dialogue by focusing on the issue of personal responsibility. If you are a parent, you might want to share this exercise with your teenager or with other parents. If you're a teenager, you can benefit by trying it with your parents and your friends.

An Exercise in Placing Responsibility

New York API—Fifteen-year-old Jennie Smith died early this morning at University Hospital as a result of head injuries sustained in a motor vehicle accident. The incident took place at 2:30 am in front of The Upstairs Tavern. Miss Smith was reportedly crossing 39th Street with a friend when the accident occurred. The occupants of the vehicle involved, Mr. and Mrs. Stan James of Worster, were unharmed.

John Peter, bartender at the Upstairs Tavern, felt terrible. He thought the girl looked old enough to drink. "Besides," he said, "she sure seemed to be able to handle her liquor."

Sandy Allen, Jennie's friend, felt terrible. After all, she was the one who invited Jennie to go out drinking. If she hadn't encouraged Jennie to drink, maybe her friend would still be alive. She also knew that if they both had not drunk so *much,* Jennie could probably have avoided the car.

The motorist felt terrible. He had been in the midst of a heated argument with his wife and did not notice the girl darting across the street. Besides, she was wearing dark clothing.

The hospital administrator felt terrible. Due to an extensive backup in the emergency room, Jennie was not attended to for over half an hour.

The triage nurse in the E.R. felt terrible. She had been helping one of the doctors on another emergency case and just could not get to Jennie soon enough.

Jennie's high school counselor felt terrible. He had spoken to her about the company she was keeping, but perhaps not as forcefully as he might have.

Mr. and Mrs. Smith felt terrible. They couldn't believe that their daughter had been drinking in a bar, especially at 2:30 in the morning. The fact that they had been at a party all evening and thought Jennie was home added to their anguish.

THE EXERCISE

1. In a few words describe how reading this exercise made you feel. _____

   _____

   _____

   Why? _____

   _____

   _____

2. Make up one more character, place him/her in the plot, and explain in a sentence or two why this person feel terrible.

   _____

   _____

   _____

3. Decide who was most responsible for Jennie's death. Put a #1 next to that person's name. Complete the ranking by numbering the remaining individuals #2 through #9, as to their **responsibility**. (#9 is least responsible.)

   Bartender _____

   Jennie's friend _____

   Motorist _____

   Hospital administrator _____

   Triage nurse _____

   High school counselor _____

   Mr. and Mrs. Smith _____

   The character you created _____

   Jennie Smith _____

4. Use this opportunity to discuss certain health dynamics which take place in your home. For example, focus on the following, plus any other questions which occur to you.

- Do adults and children in your family feel comfortable discussing alcohol, drugs and sex? If not, why?
- To what extent are you (or the children/parents) influenced by friends?
- As a parent, do (or would) you encourage discussion, negotiation, and feedback to resolve conflict with your children, or do (or would) you tell them the way things have to be, without encouraging dialogue?
- To what extent do the adults in the family act as role models for wellness?
- Do people sometimes act in a manner inconsistent with their teachings?

It is not easy to assign responsibility for another person's fate. We believe very strongly that Jennie is the individual most responsible for her fate in this made-up story—which really does happen in the real world every day. As to the others—friends, parents, school counselors—individual value systems influence our choices. There is no single best ranking, once you place a #1 next to Jennie's name.

Conclusion

Do you agree with our outlook on self-responsibility? How much consensus did you notice among those with whom you are in close and valued relationships? Are issues like this O.K. to discuss? Do you think that such discussions promote or inhibit Q.T.?

Wellness for Seniors

Growing Better—Living Fuller

There is an enormous amount of material on all the problems encountered in aging. Why has there been so little attention to the success stories? Of course the answer is society's bias toward illness and its neglect of seniors. Happily, you share our interest in countering this insidious pattern.

We have already discussed expectations—and how there is a direct plug linking the switch of beliefs to the light of results. If that sounds theoretical, let's call on George Burns to make the point in a more entertaining manner.

Asked if he believed sexual performance diminished with age, he replied: "It isn't true that just because you grow old you can't have sex. I haven't given it up, but I'm not as good as I used to be. Nobody pays me anymore." (Wall Street Journal, 10/29/79, p. 27.)

Yet the stresses and strains that accompany growing older must be acknowledged if they are to be overcome. Fears occasioned by retirement, physical changes, the loss of friends, and so on, are serious matters. Let's look closer at a few of these.

Retirement

Many people who long to retire while still on the job find that when retirement comes, it is "a fate worse than working." The leisure activities that seemed so attractive from the perspective of the workaday world sour quickly without the meaning, value and companionship that came with the job. Without continued involvement in some kind of meaningful activity—be it volunteer work, a second career, or a well-organized special project—retirement can become an empty shell.

Maintaining a cheerful outlook on life in such circumstances is difficult; post-retirement depression, in fact, is almost predictable unless careful preparations are made to prevent it.

Right or wrong, mandatory retirement is a fact of American life. If you or your spouse is soon to retire, the first thing to realize is that retirement means new work opportunities, not an end to employment. There are many kinds of work opportunities open to the retired person who is willing to explore new options and to plan well in advance. From a wellness standpoint, it is not *what* you do that is important so long as you do *something:* something with meaning for you, something that is challenging and fulfilling. Hans Selye has written that there is nothing wrong with retirement, so long as it does not interfere with your work.

When you do approach retirement, expect the event to bring a special kind of stress. Big changes in your normal routine will be stressful, and for someone who has spent the better part of a lifetime actively working, retirement will be a big change. If you believe you are being "sent out to pasture," the transition could be painful and upsetting. Nobody needs that.

Even when you reach the old age of 105 or 117.5, do not expect that you will no longer be able to work, or that you will no longer have anything to contribute to society. Grandma Moses illustrated an edition of *'Twas The Night Before Christmas* when she was 100 years old—and she didn't start painting until she was seventy-nine! Examples of equally dramatic achievements by older

persons in other fields abound. Retirement, therefore, is only a state of mind—
and presently not a very healthy one at that. A certain amount of slowing down
is perfectly natural, but an abrupt end to all work is not. Stay active, stay alert,
and stay busy—and leave the "pasture" to contented cows.

Fear of Senility

For those approaching old age, there is no fear greater than that of being
handicapped, and no handicap more threatening than the loss of one's mental
faculties. Losing your memory, your mind, or "going senile", however, is not
a very likely occurrence, statistically speaking. Fewer than 1 percent of the
population over 65 have mental disorders caused by irreversible brain damage.
Such beliefs, while false, are also medically dangerous, as negative images have
a way of becoming self-fulfilling prophesies.

There are, of course, certain degenerative diseases of the brain which afflict
old people. But senility is *not* an inevitable consequence of growing old.

This point is often lost on doctors and other health professionals as well as
laymen. When a young person forgets his coat or loses his car keys, he's being
forgetful. When a seventy-five year old does the same, he or she is going senile.
And even when there are signs of mental disorder, what the doctor diagnoses
as "senility" may actually be the byproduct of anemia, malnutrition, infection
or other problems. But since everyone expects senility in older people, premature judgments often take place.

The facts* are that only 5 per cent of the elderly are in institutions at any
one time, and the average admission age is 80. In Canada, 7 to 9 per cent of
people 65 and over are in institutions. Therefore, most people over 65 are living
and functioning in the community, not vegetating in nursing homes.

Declining Health

Disabling disease or injury is no fun at any age, but for seniors health problems often add an increased dimension of concern. Fears relating to loss of
independence, permanent disability, or frequent discomfort arising from health
problems can become a problem even before any actual sickness or injury occurs.

In a study conducted at Duke University more than half of the physical
decline in a group of elderly was "due to boredom, inactivity and the awareness
that infirmity is expected."

*Source: The Toronto Globe and Mail, February 11, 1982, p. T1.

There is nothing to be said for declining health at any time in life. Therefore, resolve to postpone such unpleasantness as long as possible! You are not helpless in this regard; we are absolutely convinced that a wellness lifestyle will dramatically reduce your prospects of illness while increasing your prospects for well-being.

Inactivity ages both the brain and the body. Staying active in civic affairs, politics, education, and social activities can help maintain vigor and health. Here are some possibilities—add some ideas of your own:

—Home repair and yard work
—Senior employment agencies
—Old-young projects—e.g., foster grandparents
—Communal purchasing
—Self-help groups
—Senior social centers
—Chapters of AARP, Gray Panthers, etc.
—College and University Programs (free or discounts)
—Community outreach, bookmobiles, nutrition mobiles
—Community health fairs
—Senior rates at entertainment

Sex

The older you get, the more you know. After all, God gave us memories so we could have roses in winter, as one poet put it. It's bad enough that young people think "old" (after age 40) people lose their interest in sex as they age; it is unacceptable for those affected to believe such rubbish.

There are changes with aging, but they are less dramatic than many of us have been led to expect. In some ways we actually get better as we age, though the following generalizations apply to most:

• spontaneous erections occur less frequently (Who needs them?)
• ejaculation takes longer due to a lowering of hormonal levels
• fertility is reduced or eliminated (e.g., females at menopause)
• otherwise, expect a receding hairline, the disappearance of a few cells, stiff tissues, lower body temperature, and a mixture of slowed chemical reactions—nothing to worry about!

Old age touches all of us fortunate enough to achieve it. Change cannot be avoided. What we can control is the way we respond and adapt. From our perspective, the initiative-filled wellness approach looks a great deal more attractive than the defensive, reactive posture. We are confident you agree.

Moving Out of the Home

There are many reasons why older people sometimes feel pressured to find a new home: difficulty in getting around, problems in keeping up a household, increasing taxes, inability to take care of oneself alone, tensions with in-laws, and others. Whatever the reason, preparation and the adoption of a positive perspective on the entire process will keep you from experiencing distress.

If staying in your home is important to you, and a financial possibility, you will need to explore various options for outside help and support well in advance of your actual needs. Everything from home health care to routine household maintenance is available if you anticipate future needs and make plans to meet them.

If you are forced to move before you are ready to do so, know that it is important to avoid a total break from the past. Familiar furniture, art, or kitchenware may not seem too valuable in your old home, but such objects take on added importance if they become your daily connection to past years. (The same point, incidentally, can be made about old and familiar friends. Many retirement dreams that involve relocation have fallen flat because old friends are simply hard to replace.)

The Loss of Loved Ones

According to stress researcher Thomas Holmes, M.D., the death of a spouse is the most stressful thing that can happen to most people. An entire pattern of life suddenly collapses, the pain of personal loss is great, and the shock of suddenly being left alone is staggering. Small wonder that all surviving spouses—at all ages—are considered more vulnerable to serious health problems for an entire year after the loss.

All older marriage partners should do what they can for the surviving partner's future. Arrange for financial matters to operate smoothly (automatically, if possible) during mourning. Share important and even trivial information that will become necessary for the surviving spouse (location of papers, keys, business procedures, details of household maintenance, and all the rest). You may want to contact a local hospice group or similar endeavor offering group support.

There is no way to make mourning painless; experiencing emotions of despair, grief, and anger is not only normal, but necessary. A formal period of mourning is a time-honored and healthy response. Know that life can and will go on—and resolve to make the most of it.

Summary

Wellness at home encompasses many things, given the role of the home as the main computer, scripting center, transition point, and so on. Relationships, communications, quality time, role expectations, and dealing with kids are among the principal concerns and issues in this dimension. In dealing with everyone, from teens to seniors, the key wellness areas (e.g., nutrition/fitness) have special applications and possibilities. Our purpose has been to encourage you to make some of these connections, and to anticipate wellness possibilities at home and elsewhere.

Chapter
5

Wellness at Work

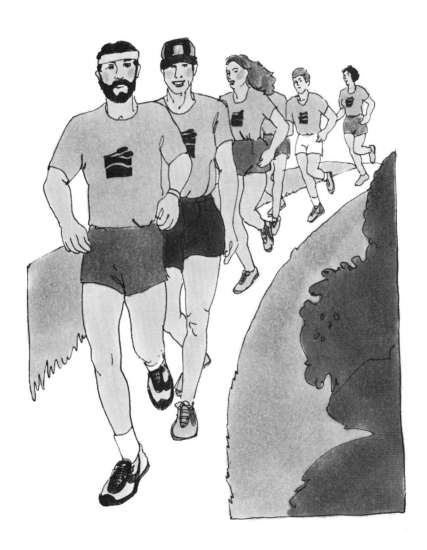

David Shelton felt good about his decision. The CEO of a highly profitable young software company, Shelton was personally enthusiastic about the 8,000 square foot fitness center which would be constructed in the new plant at a cost of $75,000. He held high hopes that it would improve employee health and morale, and hopefully boost productivity. Besides, his company would be the only one in the area with an in-house fitness center. "Who knows," he mused, "it might even help us recruit some bright young engineers from the Bay Area."

Harry Teaborn, President of Precision Manufacturing, wrestled with his decision for several weeks. After all, sixty-five percent of his assembly line workers had signed the memo asking for a shower and locker room area in the plant. "If they only knew how costly it really would be," he pondered. Rough estimates came to $5,000. (Besides, space was at a premium.) How could he justify the expenditure when he had just asked all departments to cut their budgets by 12 percent?

A decade ago, issues such as these rarely reached the attention of upper management. For the majority of U.S. companies, policies regarding employee health were clear-cut. Individual health was the employee's responsibility. The company's role was to provide a safe work environment, adequate job training, and a benefit package for disability and sickness. In 1970, American business and industry could afford this position. Times have changed.

The last decade witnessed an unprecedented rise in health care expenditures. In the preceding three years alone, our total spending as a nation for health care has mushroomed from 192 billion dollars (in 1978) to over 300 billion (in 1982).

For American business, which bears 23 percent of this burden, these figures are a great concern. Rising health care costs, along with sagging productivity, an ailing economy, and declining employee health, have mobilized many business leaders to change their philosophy regarding employee health. The question is no longer *whether* health management is a corporate responsibility—the issue has become *how* to promote better employee health and reduce health care expenditures.

Most business leaders are familiar with the well-publicized activities of Fortune 500 Companies such as Xerox, IBM, Sentry Corp., and Kimberly-Clark. These corporations provide their employees with elaborate fitness facilities and comprehensive, medically supervised risk reduction programs. Often the capital expenditure for the facilities alone is in the range of 2–4 million dollars.

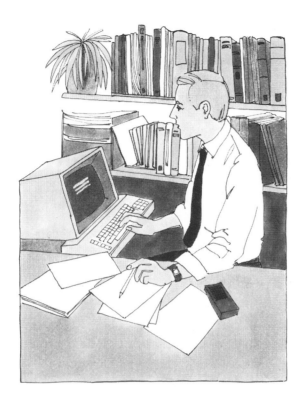

The numbers of employees who participate in these programs are impressive. The Campbell Soup Company in Camden, New Jersey, has monitored the blood pressure of their 10,000 employees since 1968 and developed in-house treatment programs to reduce the cost of care. New York Telephone provides "Health Care Management" for 80,000 employees in 1,237 locations, emphasizing health promotion classes as well as detailed history and physical exams. Ford Motor Company conducts a cardiovascular risk intervention program at four plant sites for 2,200 of its 5,500 employees.

Reading such statistics in the popular business magazines, it's all too easy for managers of smaller companies to come away with the misguided impression that promoting better employee health is a great idea but one which costs too much.

A wellness program at the workplace is a good investment at any time; but given current economic conditions, it is an absolute necessity. It is not just the high cost of medical care and accompanying escalation of health insurance rates that leads us to this conclusion. Nor is it the fact that employee illness is so damaging in terms of absenteeism, turnover, and lost productivity—and often so unnecessary. These are problems, to be sure. However, the *major* condition which a wellness program at the work site can help overcome is the downward spiralling attitudes brought on by a shrinking economy. These include fewer jobs, less job security, and deep-felt anxieties about lagging sales and other economic slowdowns and such psychological maladies as tedium, burnout, carelessness, and indifference. These conditions in turn lead to unacceptable turnover rates, poor job performance, more employee grievances, stricter supervisoral controls, frequent on-the-job accidents, and so it goes.*

Given these circumstances, described as "new rules," the "third wave," or by a variety of other terms,** most employers can no longer satisfy worker demands for a steady rise in pay. They cannot rely on purely economic incentives. The realities facing employers and employees in the present climate of hard fiscal times demands *other* than monetary satisfactions.

What do workers want, and how can a wellness program address such requirements?

According to the experts cited, workers want more than pay for their labors. They want work that is interesting, that offers opportunities for participation in decision-making, and that provides variety and informality. They also seek outlets for their creativity, the chance to assume self-responsibility, and the opportunity for goal-setting. Furthermore, they want to work in small groups—in relationships that are collegial rather than heirarchical. They want feedback—a running commentary on how they are doing. Finally, they want psychological as well as financial incentives.

Is this all feasible? Can a *job* deliver such returns? Of course not! But the workplace can, and therein rests the key to the real value of wellness at work. Producing widgets may be a bore, but coming to the place where widget production takes place can be occasion for a rewarding experience. This is the goal of a wellness program at the workplace.

This is why, under current conditions, wellness at work represents a great deal more than individualized opportunities for physical fitness and psychological/emotional well-being—and more than a personal quest for self-fulfillment. Make no mistake—these ends are worthy enough in themselves . . . but today there is more to be gained.

---

*A recent Yankelovich survey dramatizes the problem: "Twenty-seven percent of workers polled were so ashamed of the quality of the product they produced that they themselves would not want to buy it."

**See Landon Y. Jones, *Great Expectations: America and the Baby Boom Generation* (New York: Ballentine Books, 1981); Michael, Maccoby, *The Leader: Beyond the Gamesman, Managing the Workplace,* (New York: Simon and Schuster, 1981); Richard T. Pascale, *The Art of Japanese Management: Applications for American Executives* (New York: Simon and Schuster, 1981); Alberto Villoldo, and Ken Dychtwald, eds; *Millennium: Glimpses Into The 21st Century* (Boston: Houghton-Mifflin, 1981); and Daniel Yankelovich, *New Rules: Searching for Self Fulfillment In A World Turned Upside Down* (New York: Random House, 1981).

Wellness at work is nothing less than a breeding ground for worker satisfaction, raised productivity and, over time, social and economic advances. They are, in Paul Goodman's phrase from *Growing Up Absurd,* an antidote for "a high standard of living of low average quality!"

The health problems American business and industry face today are enormous:

- Premature deaths cost American industry more than $25 billion and 132 million workdays of lost production each year.

- Heart attacks kill more than one-half million Americans every year, many in their prime productive years. The American Heart Association estimates that industry pays $700 million each year just to recruit their replacements.

- Back pain afflicts about 75 million workers and accounts for $1 billion in lost output, plus $250 million in Worker's Compensation claims. Most back pain is a consequence of neglected muscles.

- People in poor condition are ill more often and recover more slowly.

- Given a "typical" company of 1,000 employees, 330 will be cigarette smokers, 160 will have high blood pressure and 100 will have alcohol or drug problems.

- Chronic fatigue and lethargy increase the risk of accidents, while efficiency and productivity sag.

Wellness Programs: The Ingredients

Sure it's great to have an elaborate in-house fitness facility, a medical director and a sizeable health care budget, but these are *not* essentials. Any company willing to actively investigate the possibility of improving employee health can devise a set of effective strategies.

A well-organized fitness program, including a modest facility, is within the reach of most U.S. corporations—especially given the willingness of employees to contribute to the cost. Thousands of U.S. companies have set aside space and provided equipment for these purposes.

Even when fitness facilities are not readily available, there are still ways to capitalize on the talent, interest and resources of the employees themselves.

Two years ago, Victor Stevens, Ph.D., a psychologist at the Kaiser-Permanente Health Services Research Center in Portland, Oregon, began charting his weekly exercise habits on a sheet of graph paper. As a reminder to stay with his program, Stevens hung the graph paper on the wall in his office. Today more than two-thirds of the 19 employees in his work unit have colorful graphs on their walls, on which they monitor their own exercise, nutrition and relaxation behaviors. The upshot is not only better health for each employee, but the creation of an environment which supports good health habits.

"The social support is the key," cites Stevens. "It's really the untapped potential which gets overlooked by those who equate health promotion with dollar amounts."

On-the-job support groups, such as the one at the Kaiser-Permanente Health Services Research Center, have been shown to help employees maintain long-lasting behavior changes such as weight reduction and increased exercise.

In an attempt to better manage their human resources, companies today are increasing their efforts in one or more of three areas:

(1) Educational programs which promote healthier employee lifestyles. These programs usually address fitness, nutrition awareness, stress management, and risk reduction. One form might be a campaign which emphasizes awareness and skill building; a comprehensive intervention program designed to reduce high-risk behavior is another. Stop-smoking and weight-loss programs are examples of the most common behavioral change programs. The goal of these programs is to reduce the staggering costs associated with lifestyle-related conditions.

(2) Early detection and treatment of disease. These programs fall under the heading of "preventive medicine" and include blood pressure, cancer, and occupational health screenings. The rationale is that with early detection, less expensive forms of treatment are called for, and longevity is enhanced.

One type of screening which has become popular over the last decade is risk-factor identification. Risk factors consist both of personal habits—for example, cigarette smoking or excessive consumption of alcohol—and medical conditions such as high blood pressure or high serum cholesterol. Identifying and quantifying personal risk factors is often the starting point for developing a personal health management program. Recently, a number of computerized health-risk appraisals have been developed and marketed throughout the United States and Canada. These printouts provide an individual with a statistical analysis of his or her probability of developing a number of diseases based on such factors as lifestyle, heredity, environment and past medical history. They compare the individual with the national average and make suggestions for increasing longevity. Health-risk appraisals are, to some extent, controversial; while some researchers have found them to be excellent tools for lifestyle assessment, others question their reliability. They usually focus on disease states and hazards, and are at best only as good as the follow-up which accompanies them. Screening programs are generally popular with employees, who appreciate the convenience of such opportunities at the worksite. One of the drawbacks of such programs is the fact that a large number of employees must be examined before a problem is found, a consideration that throws into question the cost/benefit return on each examination.

(3) Programs which encourage employees to learn medical self-care skills such as the appropriate use of health care services, back injury prevention and first aid.

Limiting the level of participation in and effectiveness of these efforts, however, is our current system of health insurance. The current system for protecting oneself (and one's family) against the potentially ruinous high costs of medical care and hospitalization leaves much to be desired. The system does not succeed in controlling or even moderating costs, improving health, or in generating employee satisfaction with company health benefit programs. For one thing, there is no incentive for avoiding or minimizing illness. There are no "payoff" mechanisms to encourage personal responsibility for health. Finally, our health insurance system does nothing to teach people the skills and techniques required for advanced states of well-being.

Most illness services are paid for by a "visa card" system. This amounts to care on the installment plan, or instant credit—no need to save to buy, no need to scrutinize the vendors or shop around for a better deal. Access to health services, whether needed or not, has become another of our forms of instant gratification.

To be sure, the present system of health insurance has certain advantages that balance the problems outlined above. It is familiar to most people—the public accepts it. It is generally well-administered by competent third-party organizations, such as Blue Cross/Blue Shield, HMOs, self-funded groups, and others. Most importantly, it spreads the risks: those with serious health problems pay less than their fair share of true costs by virtue of integration into a large pool of insured, most of whom make minor demands on the care-giving apparatus (doctors, hospitals). Of course, this is not such a great advantage for those who, either through good heredity, fortune, and/or lifestyle habits, get sick less often, since they pay the same health insurance premiums and thus support the more frequently ill. Still, many would argue that this leveling effect serves society as a form of distributive justice, with the strong aiding the weak. Finally, the current system disguises the high cost of care for salaried workers who enjoy generous health insurance benefit plans (e.g., unionized workers). Though these costs are passed along to all consumers in the form of higher prices for goods and services, they are not immediately evident at the marketplace where medical transactions occur (i.e., doctor's offices, hospitals). Again, this is a somewhat dubious advantage. Some question whether it is a good thing to anesthetize the consumer against rising medical and hospital costs.

It is in the interest of both employees and individual purchasers of health insurance to seek reforms in the current system. Such reforms must encourage, reinforce, and reward attitudes and practices which will enable people to stay well in the first place.

New Kinds of Incentives

Given the importance of wellness program at the workplace, what kind of guidelines can be suggested that will have the desired effects of encouraging personal responsibility and holding down medical costs? Here are a few:

- Modify benefit programs, especially health insurance payment policies, to reward employee *participation* in worksite wellness opportunities.
- Design the company effort in accord with established standards for wellness programming (see the elements described in Section One).
- Reward employees with financial paybacks if their health status improves (e.g. improved vital signs, less absenteeism, reduced use of medical care, or other agreed-upon measures).

These and similar incentives promise to motivate employees to investigate the deeper meanings of personal health while saving the employer substantial sums of money. Such health-promoting policies do more than just reward good health; they also support full vitality and self-determination as norms of a healthier culture.

Getting a Wellness Program Started

A wellness program is an organized approach for gaining essential attitudes, knowledge, and skills to better manage your health. The worksite can provide a long-term solution to the most difficult part of a wellness program—namely, maintenance.

A worksite wellness program has to make employees an offer they can't refuse. It does so by providing opportunities and incentives. But it must also change the work "culture" to the point where health-related activities and attitudes become the norm.

A wellness program cannot be viewed as an isolated event. It must be integrated with the policies and procedures of the organization. Unless the company's overall attitude and activities are supportive of the wellness program, it is doomed to failure.

Let's look at a few different attitudes and activities and see if you can identify your company's present work culture.

To what extent does each statement describe you and your work situation? Circle the number which corresponds to your answer.

Company Attitude	That Is Where I Work	Sometimes True	Never Applicable
If they could get a machine to replace me, they would	5	3	1
The company demonstrates a philosophy that people are important.	1	3	5
My input is valued by my superiors.	1	3	5
The company considers the quality of the work environment in policy decisions.	1	3	5
The management thrives on cut-throat competition, backstabbing, and gossip.	5	3	1
Decisions affecting my welfare are made without my opinion, advice, or consent.	5	3	1

Company Activities	That Is Where I Work	Sometimes True	Never Applicable
I feel that I am part of a team.	1	3	5
There's a spirit of playing together in my work group as well as working together.	1	3	5
When I need to calm myself I can close my eyes and relax for five minutes without people thinking I'm goofing off.	1	3	5
It's acceptable to give a desk-bound fellow worker a two-minute neck and shoulder massage.	1	3	5

Now total the numbers you have circled.   TOTAL _____

Interpretation

We know that it is not polite to call people (or collections of people) pejorative names, but this time we are going to anyway. *Sua culpa.* We have listed some descriptive terms corresponding to the point totals in the above exercise. These terms reflect the degree to which a company may be receptive to a wellness program.

My company is:

a jungle   50 points

insensitive

rigid   33 points

unimaginative

average	25 points
innovative	
progressive	17 points
enlightened	
a veritable garden for wellness	10 points

One fact about this wellness business is that the people who need health enrichment the most are often the most resistant to making lifestyle changes. So it is with companies. It seems that the heavyweight offenders (jungles, etc.) who would most benefit by an organized approach to changing the work culture are the most resistant to doing so.

Take heart if you work for a company which scored in the grim zone. Things were much worse 100 years ago! You simply have to be a bit more persuasive and clever in your approach. We will try to help you, before you have to resort to putting your resume in order. Here are some suggestions.

1. **Familiarize yourself with the facts.** First, make sure you are up-to-date about wellness before you try to sell it. It would not hurt to be familiar with the books listed in the Resource section of this guidebook. You should, for instance, be able to communicate how a wellness program is different from traditional employee benefit packages. Make good use of information about existing wellness programs at the worksite. Get the facts regarding costs and benefits. Write or call the following resource groups for invaluable assistance in this regard.

- Washington Business Group for Health
  922 Pennsylvania Ave. SE
  Washington, D.C. 20003 (202) 547-6644
- Center for Health Promotion, American Hospital Association
  840 N. Lakeshore Dr.
  Chicago, IL 60601 (312) 280–6000
- American Association of Fitness Directors in Business and Industry
  c/o President's Council on Physical Fitness
  Washington, D.C. 20201 (202) 755–7478

- Office of Health Information, Promotion and Physical Fitness
  200 Independence Ave. SW, Rm. 721B
  Washington, D.C. 20201   (202) 472–5370
- United States Chamber of Commerce
  1615 H St. NW
  Washington, D.C. 20062   (202) 659–6000
- President's Council on Physical Fitness and Sports
  Washington, D.C. 20201   (202) 755–7478

There are other sources of information, but these will give you up-to-date information on which companies have wellness programs, how much they cost, what benefits have been experienced, and similar details which your management will expect.

2. **Identify the decision-makers and convince them.** Who should you share these ideas with? Whose support will be critical in getting a program off the ground? To begin with, discuss your ideas with your immediate manager. Beyond your manager, there are several other key groups which will always play a pivotal role in supporting or undermining a program affecting the health of employees. These groups are:

- the personnel or human resources department
- the medical department
- department of occupational health and safety

Demonstrate to these people that you've done your homework. Then help them become as informed as you are. Set it up so that it is not just your idea any more. Be prepared to allow others to take the lion's share of the credit. Remember, you are interested in a program, not the glory.

Here's a thumbnail sketch of the potential which a wellness program holds for your company.

- It creates a climate where people feel and act as if they are accountable for their health.
- Productivity, employee morale, creativity are enhanced.
- Employee turnover, disability and sickness leave are reduced.
- Medical care utilization and costs are minimized.
- Employees perceive wellness activities as a means whereby the company actively cares for their health.
- Health-minded employees and family members perceive the programs as a well-deserved benefit.

3.

Survey employee interests. Next, you will require some measurement of the needs and interests of your co-workers. Encourage the personnel/human resources department to survey the work force. Try a simple questionnaire. Here's one we've used.

A Wellness Quiz

1. In general how would you rate your health?
   Excellent ☐   Good ☐   Fair ☐   Poor ☐

2. How would you rate your body weight?
   Underweight ☐   About normal weight ☐
   Slightly overweight ☐   Quite overweight ☐

3. Do you currently smoke cigarettes?
   Yes ☐   No ☐

4. Do you engage in a regular (at least 3 times a week) fitness program consisting of vigorous activity such as brisk walking, jogging, cycling, skiing, jumping rope, or aerobic dance?
   Yes ☐   No ☐

5. Do you presently belong to a fitness center?
   Yes ☐   No ☐

6. Are you satisfied with the availability and quality of the food offered at our company?
   Yes ☐   No ☐

7. Have you attempted any of the following during the past 12 months? (Check which applies)
   ☐ Losing weight   ☐ Increasing exercise
   ☐ Quitting smoking   ☐ Managing stress
   ☐ Improving nutritional habits ☐ Other health behavior change
   ☐ Reducing alcohol intake

8. If you were interested in one of the classes listed below which would take place at our company, how willing would you be to contribute time and money if necessary?

Yes, I'm interested in

☐ Losing Weight
    ☐ but only if on company time
    ☐ on my time if necessary
    ☐ only if free or paid by company
    ☐ I would be willing to pay if necessary

☐ Quitting Smoking
    ☐ but only if on company time
    ☐ on my time if necessary
    ☐ only if free or paid by company
    ☐ I would be willing to pay if necessary

☐ Reducing Alcohol
    ☐ but only if on company time
    ☐ on my time if necessary
    ☐ only if free or paid by company
    ☐ I would be willing to pay if necessary

☐ Increasing Exercise
    ☐ but only if on company time
    ☐ on my time if necessary
    ☐ only if free or paid by company
    ☐ I would be willing to pay if necessary

☐ Managing Stress
    ☐ but only if on company time
    ☐ on my time if necessary
    ☐ only if free or paid by company
    ☐ I would be willing to pay if necessary

☐ Improving Nutritional Habits
    ☐ but only if on company time
    ☐ on my time if necessary
    ☐ only if free or paid by company
    ☐ I would be willing to pay if necessary

☐ Other _____
    ☐ but only if on company time
    ☐ on my time if necessary
    ☐ only if free or paid by company
    ☐ I would be willing to pay if necessary

9. The best time for me to engage in a wellness program is (check one)
Before work ☐   Lunch Break ☐   After work ☐

10. What is the maximum amount you would be willing to pay for health classes each week?

_____ dollars

11. If you decided to make a major change in your lifestyle, how successful do you think you would be?
Very successful ☐   Moderately successful ☐   Not at all ☐

12. If you were very successful in making a major change in your health behavior, how much difference do you think it would make in your life?
Quite a lot of difference ☐   Some difference ☐   Very little difference ☐

13. Given your knowledge of our company's resources, how else might we as employees create a healthier work environment?

_____

_____

_____

_____

With data from a significant part of the work force, you have a clear picture of interest levels, a sense of the degree of commitment under varying conditions, a knowledge of priority topics, and other data which management will consider critical. Now you can move to the next stage.

4. **Establish a wellness task force.** A well-known politician once described the giraffe as an animal designed by a task force. Most task forces, it seems, keep minutes and waste hours. Here are some guidelines for making your task force an efficient one:

• Set clear goals and responsibilities. What, specifically, do you want to accomplish? Who is going to call meetings, arrange for space, circulate information, etc.?

• Develop a network of key employees to support the program.

• Plan the information flow. This includes such promotion as logos, posters, T-shirts, bulletin boards, newsgrams, articles in the company paper, letters to family members, and other available channels.

- Take advantage of the new video technology. This becomes increasingly important in decentralized organizations in which an inequality of opportunities can further exacerbate what some employees perceive as the "Ivory Tower Syndrome." Taking advantage of an already existing video capability in the bank's 200 branches, Tom Herburger, Assistant V.P. for Staff Training at U.S. Bancorp, Portland, Oregon, has included a monthly "Wellness Report" in the company's in-house video program. The video spots are supplemented with handouts providing additional health promotion material. Herburger conceived the plan as a way to "provide timely health information to all of (our) 6,000 employees." As for his hopes for the program, he adds, "When you are dealing with an organization of this size, small improvements in productivity, absenteeism and illness—even in the range of one to three percent—add up to big dollars."

- Identify community resources. Wherever you are, there is probably an individual or group with the knowledge or skills to conduct training programs in wellness. In many communities, established businesses created expressly for this purpose can be tapped. To find who they are, how much they cost, and what they do, contact such groups as the YMCA and YWCA, local hospitals with health promotion programs, doctor and nurse groups, fitness clubs, university extension divisions, and the like.

- Determine what the program will cost and where funds can be obtained. Your wellness questionnaire should provide you with a clear sense of how much money employees could be expected to contribute under favorable conditions.

5. **Introduce workshops on the wellness concept and its practical applications.** It is important for people to get the big picture. Encourage employees to develop personal wellness plans and support groups.

One of the most effective ways employees can follow up introductory lectures is by forming behavior self-management groups. These groups consist of between six and twenty-five members who meet once a week, often over a lunch period. The purpose of the meeting is to support each other by having participants compare notes on how each is progressing (e.g., losing weight, exercising more, or finding additional free time for relaxation). Usually, each person in the group keeps a log of his/her progress.

As mentioned earlier, group members can post their charts on a wall near their desks as a reminder, a reinforcement, and a record of their commitments to their own wellness and to the group that wants to support them. Several blank pieces of graph paper are included at the end of this guidebook for those who would like to begin charting their progress.

Behavior self-managment groups are inexpensive to organize and run. Furthermore, the participants themselves can become in-house facilitators, leading groups for other employees.

The social support which arises as a result of this health-oriented communication is invaluable in enabling participants to reach their individual goals. It also improves the work climate by developing teamwork, enhancing morale, and encouraging the interchange of ideas.

Here is how Joan Barrie, a captain in the U.S. Army, went about organizing a wellness program at her worksite:

Job Satisfaction

Goal: I will devote 30 minutes per week with my staff of eight individuals in order to develop a wellness environment at work within the next 2 months.

Supportive Activities:

1. I will plan an exotic, nutritious, theme-centered potluck lunch once a month.
2. I will encourage staff to agree on a color scheme and decor for the office and to decorate collectively.
3. At least 3 times per week, coffee breaks will be devoted to some group relaxation technique directed by a staff member.
4. Once per month, a "fantasy dress code" will prevail. Staff will be encouraged to wear attire suited to their own "alter ego" at work.
5. Once per week, a group exercise will be planned and staff will be allowed time to participate in swimming, running, aerobic dance, or gymnastics.

Goal: I will encourage other department managers to learn about creating a wellness environment at work.

Supportive Activities:

1. I will include other staff in activities planned as above.
2. I will organize a fact-finding group to determine wellness needs and wellness projects for other staff personnel.
3. I will plan sessions on stress reduction and coping techniques for all staff.

To Avoid Sabotage:

1. I will review weekly progress compared to intentions.
2. I will encourage one other person each week to go to the wellness club at work.

6.

Keep track of the results. In order to get the resources to expand your program once it has been started, you have to demonstrate to management that you have achieved some success. A number of indices are available. These include:

- Demonstrated employee willingness to invest time and money in wellness programs.
- Number of employees performing regular fitness activities.
- Weight-loss and stop-smoking success rates.
- Subjective measurements of employees' ability to manage stress through increased coping and communication skills.
- Detection and effective follow-up of employees with high blood pressure and other risk indices.
- Reduction in medical claims.
- Changes in morale as determined by employee attitude or work climate surveys.
- Improvement in job performance.

Summary

The President of our mythical software company described at the beginning of this chapter took a risk based on his reading of economic and social trends. Actual companies are doing the same.

Here are a few success stories that have come our way:

- At New York Telephone Company, nine wellness programs saved the company $2.7 million last year in absence and treatment costs, "and that's an extremely conservative figure," said Dr. Loring W. Wood, the company's medical director for research and development

  These conservative estimates by New York Telephone do not include money saved by increased well-being, improved work attitude and better family relations leading to increased productivity among workers and decreased turnover, nor do they include savings in employee replacement costs or dollar figures for lives saved.

- At Canada Life Assurance Co. in Toronto, a study showed that a fitness program saved the company $36,975 in health care costs the first year. The program was so popular with employees that turnover costs also were reduced by an annual figure of $231,000.

- At Campbell Soup Co. in Camden, N.J., a colon/rectal cancer screening program saved $245,000 over 10 years. The company estimated that each case of colon/rectal cancer costs $66,000 in medical fees covered by insurance plus lost time and replacement costs if a new employee must be trained.

- Dow Chemical Co.'s Texas Division determined that smokers there (33% of the work force) averaged 5.5 days more absenteeism, 7.7 days more disability and 12% more illnesses per year than non-smokers when Dow initiated a stop-smoking program, one-quarter of its smokers quit.
- Marvin Kristein, an economist working at the National Institutes of Health in Bethesda, Md., created a model suggesting that the average white-collar company would save about $466,000 in medical costs per 1,000 employees annually by helping them reduce disease factors in their lives.
- Firestone Tire & Rubber Co. claims it has saved $1.7 million in annual savings "in just absenteeism, accident and sickness, and medical surgery costs" as a result of a comprehensive employee assistance program.
- Kennecott Corporation found that the 150 men involved in its Employee Assistance Program showed 52% better attendance on the job, a 75% cut in weekly indemnity costs and a 55% drop in health, medical and surgical costs.

Current efforts, no matter how innovative and comprehensive, are just beginnings. The workplace of the future will, in our view, be quite different from the current norm, insofar as opportunities for wellness are concerned. While settling, temporarily, for those advances that are currently possible, think ahead to these Utopian possibilities and fix your sights on them.

Chapter
6

Wellness at Play

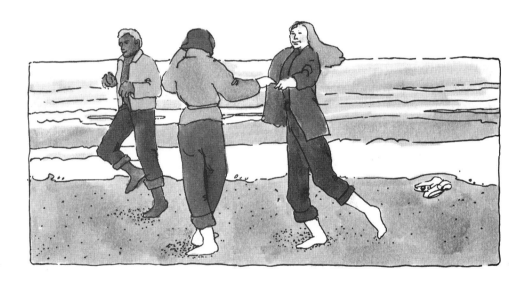

Much of what you do at play (which is loosely defined here to mean "free" time not related to family/relationship responsibilities or to functions associated with earning a living) is already targeted to the pursuit of wellness. An example would be reading this book, assuming you are not doing so because your parent/spouse or boss/associates begged you to do so. Play time is discretionary time, and these hours are loaded with opportunities for wellness.

Your capacity to have fun is influenced by many factors—some outside of your control, but most a function of how you and others have organized your life. Numerous variables affect this element of play. They include: the availability and quality of leisure time, the power of the work ethic, the nature of your parental "tapes," the kinds of friends you have, the extent to which you like yourself, and the kinds of subpersonalities with which you have to contend.

Wellness requires, and implies, the ability to have fun. What could be more important than that? So before going any further with this theoretical stuff about fun, let's test your "FQ", or "fun quotient."

How much out-and-out fun are you having in life? Check whichever statement comes closest to your situation.

_____ Life is a blast. I'm having a ball.

_____ I have a great deal of fun at times.

_____ I experience more than my share of fun.

_____ I suppose I am about average in this regard.

_____ I need to give this a little more attention.

_____ I am not having much fun at all.

_____ I am miserable.

_____ I am against the very idea of having fun. Life is a serious matter. Fun is not appropriate.

How did you do? If you checked any of the top five boxes, you're doing fine. (Congratulations if you marked one of the first three.) If you marked "not having much fun" or "miserable," this chapter is for you. If you marked the last box . . . well, maybe you'll like the next chapter.

Think of the minutes spent with these activities as an opportunity for fun. You do not have to *be* serious to *do* something worthwhile. Play occasions are in their own way reflective times. They help us see where we're heading. The exercises in this chapter will help you assess your connectedness to the rest of the world and your directions, purposes, and goals. We will look at ways in which accumulated hassles drain your energy and weaken your resolve for improving your health. We will also provide some suggestions in hopes of alleviating the harmful effects of this accumulation.

After such a workout, we thought you would be ready for a bit of relief, so we have included some instructions on how you can "win" the Boston Marathon. Next, you might enjoy trying the "unique fruit" exercise with a group of friends or testing your assertiveness in the face of low-level worseness.

Have fun.

The Beyond-Personal-Wellness Exercise

To be of service to others, it helps to have your own act together. You first help yourself, then you positively affect others. Along the way, however, you might need to assess your position on larger matters beyond the wellness dimensions of nutrition, fitness, and stress management. The way in which you relate to the world around you, to people, and to institutions may add to or detract from your overall health performance.

Please check yes or no to the following:

• My income and financial prospects are adequate; I do not have to spend what I consider excessive amounts of time concerning myself with how to manage the basics (food, shelter, clothing, and security).

Yes _____ No _____

• My life situation is reasonable as a base for wellness; specifically, my home life is not disruptive, threatening, or unsafe.

Yes _____ No _____

• I am aware of and interested in current events on national and international levels.

Yes _____ No _____

• I participate to some extent in politics, at least to the point that I usually vote, know who my representatives are, and occasionally go as far as to write a letter, place a call, or attend a meeting to express my views.

Yes _____ No _____

• I take care of myself in hazardous situations. For example, I pay heed to the location of exit doors in airplanes. I *always* wear seat belts in my car, and try to do so when riding with others. I do not dwell in places where I am likely to be in jeopardy or to feel unwelcome for any reason.

Yes _____ No _____

• I refrain from speeding, running stop signs, and taking other risks in cars.

Yes _____ No _____

• I use public transit, if possible.

Yes _____ No _____

• I conserve energy (e.g., home temperature, recycling, use of non-polluting products).

Yes _____ No _____

• I relate comfortably and well with others, belong to a club or two, and am somewhat involved with or at least supportive of some community organization.

Yes _____ No _____

• I make an effort to know my neighbors; I would surely take action (e.g., call local authorities) if I observed a hazardous condition or a crime.

Yes _____ No _____

Interpretation

Affirmative answers obviously indicate that you appreciate the need to build strong bridges to the islands around your own. A few negative responses are not a basis for judging yourself a recluse. Just consider how much easier it is to experience the highest returns from optimal health and rewarding personal performance when you share your life with others.

As usual, we probably overlooked a few items. What social issues do you consider important?

_____

_____

_____

_____

Self-Responsibility
Great Events and Little Hassles

In recent years, a lot of attention has been given to major events as the prime factors in the buildup of stress. The death of a spouse, divorce, separation, job crisis, and so on—these are among the events which can be indexed to predict your chances of becoming ill from excessive stress.

We have a different view of the stress dynamic. It seems to us that whether you do well or poorly in managing stress is determined by three variables: (1) how you respond to it; (2) the frequency or quantity of minor upsets and annoyances; and (3) the extent to which you acknowledge that you have control over the way these occurrences affect you. By taking responsibility for your reaction, you reserve for yourself the final power to determine the effect of any stress event, large or small. In the process, you automatically diminish the stress load attached to varied everyday upsets and difficulties.

Rather than explaining how this works in great detail, we'll give you this simple exercise to illustrate the idea.

The Hassle Compendium: A Cost-Benefit Exercise

Think of the stress factors that you experience more or less every day; make a list of them. Start at the beginning when you awake, and complete the list as you review the ordinary, day-in, day-out little annoyances that seem almost inevitable. Examples might include:

- rushing to leave the house on time
- doing battle with commuter traffic or crowded bus conditions
- early morning panic at work about deadlines, ringing phones, etc.
- too little time for exercise at lunch hour
- tense meetings
- lack of quiet time to get centered or rebalanced
- commute rush at end of day
- family crises upon entering the home
- noise level at dinner
- not able to locate tools in hobby room
- too tired to go out with friends for club meeting

This list of examples, of course, may not be at all comparable to the hassles you come up with. This is not the intent; the idea is just to help you get started by showing the kind of everyday stress factors which you should now attempt to identify as typical of your normal day.

Give yourself five minutes to complete this activity. Avoid the temptation to read the next part of the instructions until you have finished your hassle listing.

_____

_____

_____

_____

_____

_____

_____

_____

Interpretation

Now that you have a list of everyday hassles, upsets, or stress factors, examine each of the items to determine the *payoffs* you get from each situation.

Sound contradictory? It shouldn't. There are payoffs for almost every human activity; in one way or another, we are getting something out of everything we do. It may be money, recognition, acceptance, or attention. The problem is *we are not aware of many payoffs* because we do not take time to examine our behaviors.

Try to make a note about a payoff next to each hassle factor. Note especially those hassles that occur in and around the play portion of your day. Here are a few examples to help you get started:

Hassle	**Payoff**
rushing to leave house on time	getting to sleep fifteen minutes more
commute rush at end of day	able to live in country

Is it easy to identify what you derive from permitting a specific upset to recur on a regular basis?

Take another five minutes right now for a payoff hunt. Be fearless, creative, and open to the idea that there may be a payoff or reward of some kind for allowing any given stress event to occur day in and day out. Granted, you may not be able to find payoffs for each of your hassles, but a great many have identifiable benefits.

Five-Minute Break for the Great Payoff Quest

One woman in a recent seminar had time pressures listed as the constant hassle in all phases of her daily routine. She was a homemaker with two teen-aged children, running a part-time business, writing a novel, taking graduate course work for a master's degree, and carrying on an affair. She also was trying to read up on skydiving in preparation for a first jump scheduled within a few weeks.

Just consider all the choices being made by this person. Once she identified the payoffs, a wonderful thing happened. She realized that she *was* in control, *was* responsible for the pace and events of her life, and *was* able to decide if the stresses that resulted were excessive in relation to the goals pursued or satisfactions realized.

Which leads into your next task. Are your payoffs worthy of your hassles? Do a quick cost-benefit analysis with your list and the notes you have about payoffs. Is the balance there? Or are the hassles taking more of your energies than the satisfactions are putting back? Place an X next to the items that do not pay off sufficiently and a Y next to those that do. You can also put a question mark where the cost/benefit analysis is inconclusive.

Now comes the fun part. It's time to plan a course of action. You have about five choices. Briefly, they are:

1. Do nothing. When you acknowledge the payoffs of everyday hassles by bringing them into conscious focus, you lower your stress load. This in itself puts you ahead of the game.
2. If costs and benefits (payoffs) are out of line, think of other ways to get the benefits which the hassles provide, but at a lower cost. In most cases, there are plenty of options, if you examine the situation carefully.
3. Abandon the benefit—and terminate the activity or event that precipitates the recurring hassle. In the case noted above, the woman in the workshop decided she was overextended and, in order to lessen her stress, should give up her husband!
4. Make drastic changes in your environment. Maybe it is time for a new job, career, location, mate, or whatever.
5. Make changes in you. This is the last area most of us contemplate. It means reexamining what you want to do with your life, how you look at situations, and other considerations about the internal environment of the heart and mind.

There is another dimension to this exercise: do it with a group of your friends. You will have to assume the leader role, although you should take part to derive most from the process. Consider what you have already done by yourself as good practice for doing the same with your friends. Any number can participate, but organize your friends into groups of six. Here are the steps to follow:

1. Explain the importance of little, everyday stress events.
2. Ask each person to write a list of daily hassles. No discussion. Time limit of five minutes.
3. Divide into groups; each person mentions the hassles he/she has listed.
4. Everyone is then asked to identify payoffs, as explained above. Discuss.
5. For those unable to see any payoffs, ask others in the group for suggestions on benefits derived from what at first seem like stresses (hassles) with no redeeming qualities.
6. Have everyone look at cost/benefits, and make appropriate checks and marks.

Conclude this activity by asking people, after your explanation, what they thought about during the activity or after it was over. Encourage a sharing of ideas and feelings. You will get more out of the exercise in leading others through it, and you will be making a useful contribution to the well-being of your friends.

The "Hassle Compendium" exercise serves to illustrate a number of basics about self-responsibility and stress management. It shows vividly what really matters for better—health enrichment and effective functioning—or worse—high levels of distress leading to submarginal performance. It also demonstrates how minor hassles, which individually seem harmless, can be powerful in combination with large numbers of other hassles day after day. What is more, this process dramatizes the fact that we can all increase our control over situations by consciously examining what we derive, in one way or another, from the conditions we *choose* to permit to exist in our daily lives.

The *costs* of taking greater responsibility (e.g., the risk of failure, the time and discipline required) seem insignificant when compared with the benefits to be derived (e.g., enhanced sense of mastery, diminished stress, and expanded choices). Furthermore, the best payoff is the knowledge that you are the source and manager of life events, the satisfaction that comes from believing that you are the cause rather than the effect of your life events, large and small.

Creative Winning at Wellness

Introduction

You need *perspective* to win the Boston Marathon. You need to want to win. You need preparation and talent, and money to get there. Other helpful assets include encouragement from your friends, the right temperature, careful planning, and a generous measure of luck at avoiding injuries, police strikes, and other setbacks.

However, let's look more closely at this perspective itself. Do you realize that the time-honored, all-American focus on winning can be hazardous to your health? This no-holds barred, simplistic, and no-compromise approach to winning is based on the idea that to win is to win is to win—period. This urge, if taken literally, can be disastrous to your finances and ruinous to your spiritual well-being.

The simplistic mindset of winning as meaning first across the finish line is seen most dramatically in professional sports. Winning means taking the Super Bowl, the World Series, and the Stanley Cup—at the expense of all the rest (the "losers"). There is no in-between. This philosophy creates a lot of losers.

Naturally, the running set, blessed with an abundance of creativity, precious bodily fluids, and spectacular physiques, has led the way in loosening up the idea that winning equals being first—period. When it comes to running, we celebrate winners in abundance. We honor first man, first woman, first master male, first master female, first kid (male and female), even first male and female centipede (at the San Francisco Bay-to-Breakers). In brief, we consider winning synonymous with putting forth our best effort, as going to the edges of our limits to test a rival or ourselves. In one way or another, everyone receives his or her due; genuine homage is accorded all who participate with vigor.

The Boston Marathon offers a metaphor for the right perspective on winning.

A Creative Winning Exercise

If a rose is a rose is a rose, is it also true that to win is to win is to win? Or, to put it another way, is there more to the great American tradition of being a winner than being first? If so, does this have anything to do with wellness?

We suggest that there is a way to *win more often* with the same level of effort in a manner that provides *added satisfactions*. We call this *creative winning*.

You can be a creative winner. The technique is simple, free, pleasantly challenging, and available to everyone. Take this test. Think back to the Boston Marathon on April 21, 1981. Make a check mark (✔) after the names of the winners in each of the two divisions.

Check the Winners of the Boston Marathon*

Males

A. —Toshihiko Seko, Japan
B. —Craig Virgin, Lebanon, Il.
C. —Bill Rodgers, Stoneham, Ma.
D. —John Lodwick, Dallas, Tx.
E. —Malcolm East, Pittsburgh, Pa.
F. —All the above
G. —All the above, plus the 6,845 others participating in the event

Females

A. —Allison Roe, New Zealand
B. —Patti Catalano, West Roxbury, Ma.
C. —Joan Benoit, Exeter, NH.
D. —Jacqueline Gareau, Canada
E. —Sissel Grottenberg, Norway
F. —All of the above
G. —Same as G, other column

All answers are potentially correct, depending on your perspective on winning. Seko and Roe were the first of their genders to cross the finish line, but surely others won too. The next four were quoted as having been pleased with their respective performances, and the thousands who finished after the elite few were ecstatic about the event. So, in another sense, there were many, many winners. They had shared in the experience of testing their limits in the most historic, colorful, and exciting foot race in the world. They had "done Boston!"

Isn't this a happy contrast to the professional sports mentality that represents victory as a conquest over others, as a pinnacle large enough for only one, and as an all-or-nothing proposition? It opens up all kinds of possibilities for distinguishing ourselves, especially for meeting our own personal standards.

Naturally, it takes a bit of practice to glimpse the expanded possibilities. In part, this approach was inspired by the top runners at the awards ceremony after the 85th running of the BAA's colorful and exciting extravaganza. We call it "creative winning"; at Boston, it was raised to the status of an art form. A few examples are in order.

Bill Rodgers (properly) said he won (in a fashion) by demonstrating that he could still stay with the best, break 2:11, and represent himself "honorably."

*You never heard of any of these people? Relax, neither did Mark.

He did so with his customary measure of grace, wit, dignity, and cogency—Rodgerian trademarks. Surely he is a winner.

Craig Virgin won by adding lustre to his image as America's premier racer at any distance event up to the Big One and as an articulate public relations machine. Also, he proved he could run a very fast marathon (2:10:26).

Many of the top-ranked women won (despite Allison Roe) by setting new personal records and acquiring handsome contracts with shoe companies and other entrepreneurs.

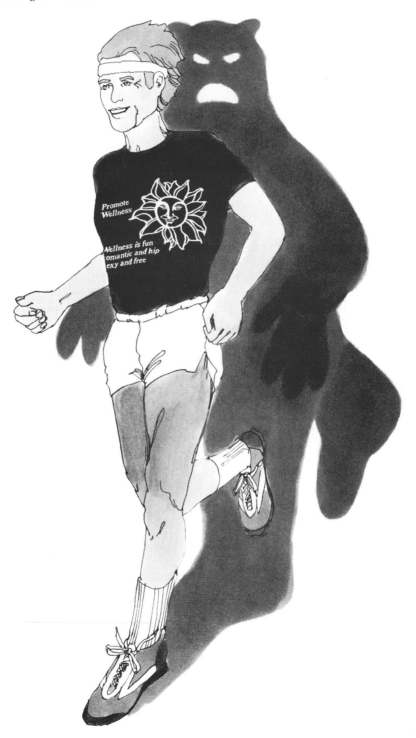

On a personal note, I (Don) would like to comment on my own performance. My goal at the 1981 Boston Marathon was to run it in approximately two hours and thirty-six minutes, a sub-six-minute-per-mile pace. I had been very close just a month earlier (2:40:18); given the excitement of the crowds lining the route and my arduous preparation (80 miles per week), I thought I could do it. I was ready. I was going to *win* by running 2:36 or better.

I was ahead of schedule at the 20-mile mark. I was *blazing a trail* to fame and glory. I felt great. I even fantasized a bit. These people were not here to cheer Seko, Virgin, Rogers, Catalano, or even John Kelley running his 50th Boston Marathon at age 73! They were here to go bananas as I passed triumphantly on my way to a 2:36 personal record. Six more miles and the word would go out to the Universe: Ardell has done it! I could taste it. Shoe companies, candy manufacturers, and hamburger chains would seek my endorsement of their products. Johnny Carson would beg me to appear on his show! The Mayor, the governor, and even Bill Rodgers would want to shake my hand. No wonder I was smiling and waving to my fans.

Tragically, an invisible Bigfoot leaped on my legs at the 22-mile mark. In the space of about a block, my pace went from 5:55 to, at best, 10 minutes per mile. In two blocks, it slowed down to become measurably only in glacial terms. My legs locked with cramps, I was a one-man traffic jam. For me, the marathon was over, the fantasy shattered. No Johnny Carson show, no endorsements, no handshakes from the mayor, the governor, or Bill Rodgers. I limped into the crowd, pretended it was only sweat in my eyes, and rode a streetcar to the hotel.

Soon, however, I remembered the concept of creative winning. Sure enough, there was indeed another way to look at things. Yes, I had dropped out. I did not break 2:36. Yes, I hurt. No, not a soul would have guessed that I had won something. But thanks to creative winning, I was a champion! I won my division! A careful analysis of the results revealed (to me) that I was the first male master (over forty) runner from Northern California with blue eyes, weighing more than 170 pounds, of unattached marital status, with an unusual sense of humor, to reach the 22-mile mark. I won, in other words, by choosing the right division.

You, too, can win at whatever you do, by selecting the right division. Wellness is a wonderful division, no matter what games you play, work you do, or people with whom you share yourself.

There are but six rules for creative winning:

1. Set high but attainable expectations.
2. Do your best to achieve them.
3. Evaluate how you do.

4. If you make it, celebrate and set new, higher standards.
5. If you don't quite make it, reinterpret the goal, celebrate, and try again (be willing to modify the original expectation).
6. Be good to yourself.

When in doubt, ask this question: What point of view about the situation will serve my needs, help me move on, and get the results I desire in life? Do this and creative winning solutions will soon be evident.

Think about any recent setbacks you experienced. Try to remember some minor disappointments, some expectations or desires which seemed within reach but which, for varied reasons, did not turn out. List a number of such situations briefly, noting your goal and the outcomes.

Example: I wanted to break 2:36 in Boston. I dropped out at 22 miles.
Your situation:

1. _____
2. _____
3. _____
4. _____
5. _____

Now try the creative winning approach. How might you reinterpret these situations in light of creative winning?

Example: I ran a great 22-mile race. I enjoyed the experience. I learned a lot that will help me modify my training and racing. I think I'll set a slower pace next time.
Your situations:

1. _____
2. _____
3. _____
4. _____
5. _____

Not many are capable of beating Seko in a marathon, or starring in the World Series or Superbowl, or getting elected President of the U.S., or making millions of dollars, or otherwise gaining superstar status.

Fortunately, you do not need to pursue extremes to be winners. All that is needed is a wider perspective on winning. Good luck on this; have fun with the idea. With creative winning, you take the sting out of setbacks while safeguarding the thrill of victories. Best of all, you get to win more often.

The Unique Fruit Exercise

You know about the Hawthorne effect, right? This is another term for experimenter bias. Roughly, it means that the results of a test or study are flawed because some variable in the experimenter which was not controlled ruined the validity of the results.

To avoid the Hawthorne effect, the following exercise is introduced with no explanation. If we explained the rationale for doing this exercise, it might influence the way you perform the activity. Try it without knowing the grand plan behind the process. We will explain all—later.

Directions: Take a dozen apples, oranges, bananas, strawberries, pineapples, guavas, lemons, papayas, watermelons, grapefruits, or whatever fruit is readily available or especially appealing. Use only one kind of fruit; no mixing will work.

Pass them around to your friends, who should be arranged in a circle, seated comfortably. Ask each person to take one piece of fruit. There are eight steps involved in this activity. The first is to have each person examine his/her apple,

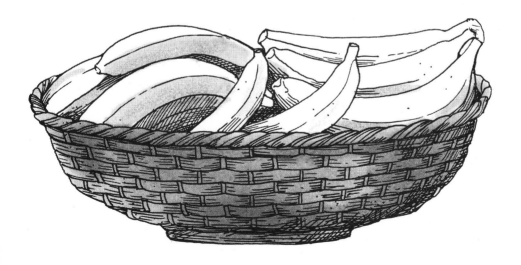

orange, or whatever. Notice the texture, color, size, contours, weight, and other special markings or characteristics of the fruit. Smell it, rub it on your chin, and otherwise proceed as a wine taster would. Notice the body clarity, and like qualities. Get sensuous with your fruit—use your imagination to "relate" to it. Pretend, for example, that it is a rifle and you are a Marine at boot camp in Paris Island. Or that it is Romeo—and you are Juliet. Contemplate that fruit! Know it intimately. After about three minutes of this (a little background music might help), move on to step two.

Step two requires that you surrender your fruit. Pass the fruit to the center of the circle. Mix them in a large bowl or whatever is available.

Step three is a relaxation pause of one minute. Each person takes several deep breaths, combined with a few silent suggestions as in self-hypnosis. The desired mood is one of relaxation, serenity, and calm.

Step four is to pass the fruit back around the circle.

Step five is for everyone to find his or her fruit. Not any fruit, but the same one he or she examined, fondled, experienced, and otherwise focused upon and related to. Keep passing the specimens until everyone is satisfied that *the* fruit belonging to him/her has been returned. This usually takes only a minute or two; people are amazed to learn that they know *exactly* which fruit is theirs!

Step six is to eat the fruit. Slowly, lasciviously, with great attention to subtleties of taste, smell, touch, feel, and after-effects.

Step seven is to ask each person to comment on the entire process. Ask people to note what thoughts they had during this activity—and now, after it. Also ask how they felt doing it. Did they notice anything unusual? Was the fruit different from usual? All comments are acceptable. Acknowledge what each person volunteers, but do not evaluate it, or inadvertently cause anyone to feel uncomfortable.

Step eight is to explain what took place.

Interpretation

We have two points to make about this little parlor game.

The first might be obvious. You can get more enjoyment from food if you slow down and pay attention. Too often we eat on the run, or eat when we are under tension, upset, or preoccupied by another activity (e.g., reading, watching TV, thinking about a problem or being somewhere else). When this happens, we miss out. We get less nutritive value from food, and we enjoy it less though we might eat more of it. All in all, unconscious dining is a poor bargain. This exercise dramatizes the alternative, and shows experientially that being aware of eating makes the process more satisfying.

The second lesson is more subtle. It is also more valuable. It is about unique-ness, individuality, and the special wonder of variations on a theme, a pat-tern—or in this case—a fruit. The implication takes us one more step to a renewed appreciation for the uniqueness of human beings.

If one special apple, orange, or other fruit can be identified in a basket of such fruit, can we not acknowledge the infinitely more diversified and rich in-dividuality that we all possess as humans? Just as your apple (or whatever) is different from every other apple, so you and everyone else in the circle are extraordinary and pricelessly unique, unlike anyone else in the universe.

You knew this anyway, of course. Sometimes, however, it is worthwhile to slow down and enjoy the flowers (and fruits), and to reflect on how special you and those whom you care about really are. Think about that next time you see an apple. Or a friend.

Helping Friends and Others Stop Smoking

No matter how wellness-oriented your lifestyle is or will become, no matter how charmed your existence may be, there are going to be times when you will be tried and tested. Cigarette smoking may do just that.

Smoking is one of those issues that divides people into two very distinct camps. Approximately two thirds of the adult population of North America presently have unadulterated lungs; the other third consumes 900 billion cigarettes each year.

These two groups do not always get along so well. In fact, when smokers and nonsmokers have to work, eat, or play together, the question of rights and privileges is often raised—sometimes vociferously, other times mutely.

There are a number of ways in which the two factions could coexist peace-fully: (**1**) All smokers could give up their habit. (**2**) All nonsmokers could take it up. (**3**) Nonsmokers could support their smoker friends' efforts to kick the habit. (**4**) A set of very strict and enforceable rules concerning public places could be enacted.

Let's take a quick look at each of these approaches.

1. All smokers could give up their habit.

It is not easy to stop smoking. Cigarettes are a smoker's best friend. They are reliable, dependable, and predictable. (How many friends do you have who consistently meet these criteria?) Smokers have grown to associate cigarettes with moments of pleasure, sorrow, joy, relaxation and relief from boredom. Cigarettes accompany mealtime, breaktime, phone conversations, ironing, television, and even showering. When you consider that the most die-hard smoker may light up between 300,000 and 500,000 times in a lifetime, you can appreciate the power of these associations. The $422 million that the tobacco industry spends on advertising each year certainly helps to reinforce the connection.

Stopping smoking is tantamount to the death of a friend. There is a period of mourning which involves both physical (short-term) and psychological (long-term) withdrawal.

There are, however, a few rays of hope on the stop-smoking horizon. The American Cancer Society, Seventh Day Adventists, local lung and heart associations, hospital wellness centers, and a number of private organizations now have well-established programs to help even the most reluctant smoker stop. Still, chances are overwhelming that option #1 will not become a reality in our lifetime.

2. All nonsmokers could take it up.

If you even entertain this notion at this point in *Planning for Wellness,* we have lost you. You would be best advised to return to the preface and start reading again.

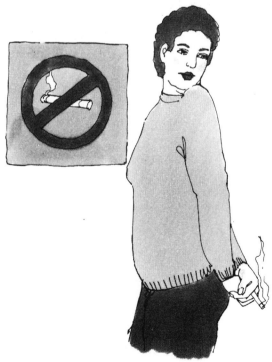

3. Nonsmokers could support their smoker friends' efforts to kick the habit.

This is an attractive possibility. It requires the patience of Buddha, the wisdom of Solomon, and the insight of Freud, but it can be done.

This kind of group approach works best at work. Smoking no longer is the smoker's problem alone—it becomes a problem for the total group to solve. To help friends stop smoking you must be both positive and thoughtful. Provide some extra TLC. You may want to reward them with a special dinner or a massage, take them to a ballgame or concert, or give them a surprise gift. Above all, remain considerate of the difficulty of their effort.

4. Rules concerning public places could be enacted.

There are two problems with method #3. First, the person needs to be a friend; second, he or she must already want to give up smoking.

All too often, nonsmokers find themselves in situations where the only way to save their lungs is an enforceable nonsmoking ordinance. Unfortunately, such legislation is proceeding at a snail's pace in most communities. Does this mean that nonsmokers need to passively accept the documented health risks of others' cigarette smoke? Or could a bit of assertiveness help make our air cleaner and safer?

The Assertiveness Exercise

Picture yourself in the following situation. It is a cool spring evening in Ft. Lauderdale. You are on a combination vacation/business trip. It has been a splendid day—ocean swimming, fresh and wholesome foods, good friends, creative moments, quiet times, exercise, successful project negotiations, the works. You are seated in a fine restaurant with a special person. All's right with the world (or at least it seems that way). You have tranquility, a positive outlook, and romance. Life is great!

And then it happens. At first, it seems the signal comes from some mysterious inner alarm. You sense, at some instinctive level, an ominous foreboding. Soon, the source becomes clear: there are smokers at the next table! They are fouling your air. Worse, the spell of enchantment and serenity seems to have been extinguished by clouds from the noxious weeds.

What are you going to do about it?

Here is a list of possibilities. Please place a check next to the statements that more or less express what action(s) you would be *likely* to take (as opposed to what you wish you had the chutzpah to do).

- I would take no action. People have a right to smoke in restaurants. Why should I impose my expectations on others? _____
- Summon the maitre d' and request seating elsewhere. _____
- Walk to the table of smokers and ask if they would kindly consider not smoking. _____
- Stride authoritatively to the table and deliver a hell-fire and damnation account of the hazards of smoking. Request that if they must smoke, to please have the decency not to exhale. _____
- Same as above, except that you add that your companion is missing her right lung and the remaining lung does not work so well, either. You might add that she had a pack-a-day habit, a subtle hint that refraining may be in their interest, also. _____
- Same as above, except that you first turn their table over as an attention-getting device before describing your friend's breathing difficulties. _____
- None of the above. These choices are either cowardly, obnoxious, self-defeating, crisis-producing, or otherwise reflective of a failed imagination. Here are a number of other possibilities. (Write a few other choices. Have some fun with this. List a few things you would fantasize doing.)

- _____

- _____

- _____

Now, place a check next to the actions you really might consider taking. Decide what your response would be in this or a similar situation.

Interpretation

The possibilities listed above span the behavior spectrum from meek passivity to out-and-out aggression.

Assertiveness implies stating your needs in a positive, pleasant and constructive manner. It involves raising sensitive issues in a way which allows the receiver of your message to actively listen and respond appropriately. By practicing assertive behavior, you build self-respect and confidence, achieve your goals, and take greater responsibility for your own well-being. Assertiveness is a win-win situation; both you and the other person come out ahead.

Aggressiveness, on the other hand, is a win-lose proposition. The aggressive person may achieve his or her desired result, but only at the expense of others. Aggressiveness is tactless, insensitive, and inappropriate. An aggressive person leaves the recipient of the action feeling angry, humiliated, resentful and devalued.

In learning to be assertive, not aggressive, it may help to anticipate situations which will challenge you to react assertively. Then you can respond in a practiced, deliberate way to circumstances that otherwise might evoke haphazard, unpredictable responses. In the situation listed above, the following four points might have helped you respond appropriately:

1. Do not allow strangers to dictate your moods and actions. You can't always decide who sits near you in restaurants, but you do not have to give whoever lands within range the power to determine whether you enjoy your meal.
2. Remember that the action you take should support the result you desire. Know what result you desire; think it through. In the above case, the desired result is to enjoy the experience of being in that restaurant at that time under these unique circumstances. Whether the offenders do or do not smoke (or talk loudly, pick their noses, pass gas, or otherwise display poor form and no class) should not be the principal concern. Your challenge, it seems, is to do what you must to be able to enjoy the meal, the setting, and your company. It *might* require that you ask the smokers not to, that you move to another table, or both—or something else.
3. Your actions should be considerate of others, and just may be of service as well. The person you are with will be observing your reactions and behavior. The people at the offending table will be affected by what you say and do. Do not assume that all smokers are neo-nazis or moral slugs. Help them to save face. Be as graceful as possible; the smokers may be reasonable people, given half a chance.
4. Anticipate this kind of problem. When you arrive at a restaurant, ask for the no-smoking section, even if you *know* they do not have one. Courteously ask that the manager be advised that patrons suggested an area be set aside for non-smokers. Ask to be seated in a remote area or section where a quick reconnaisance reveals no signs of air-polluters.

One last suggestion. Invite your friends, including a few who are smokers, to do this exercise. Have them discuss their responses, and engage them in an examination of strategies to employ for these kinds of situations. Jazz it up a bit; try variations on the theme.

Smoking is just one of the many life situations which will test your ability to be constructively assertive. Here are a few others.

• Your immediate supervisor at work has the annoying habit of compulsively whistling atonal tunes in the key of F# minor throughout the workday. You work in close proximity and find his habit distracting and annoying. What would you do?

_____ Nothing; after all, he is your supervisor and you have an important job performance review coming up soon.

_____ Find an opportune time to let your boss know that his whistling is disturbing your ability to work and discuss possible solutions to the problem.

_____ Bring a radio to work and blare loud rock music all day long.

Your solution _____

_____

_____

- Your lover has "garlic breath" after eating a large Italian dinner (and not brushing thereafter). You are in a tender embrace whispering terms of endearment to one another. The atmosphere is right, but your friend's offensive breath is dampening your amorous mood and stifling your romantic intentions. You would:

  _____ Ignore your nose. Sidestep the bad breath by concentrating on other areas of your friend's anatomy.

  _____ Ask if there are any garlic bread leftovers. After all, if you don't want to fight 'em, join 'em.

  _____ Begin a short monologue on the merits of fluoride as a cavity fighter in today's toothpaste. Then casually mention how great Crest both tastes and smells. Besides, you just so happen to have an extra toothbrush in the bathroom.

  _____ Suggest that you both go brush your teeth prior to going any further in your love-making pursuits.

Your solution: _____

_____

_____

- You are spending the day with an old acquaintance who has acquired the noxious habit of swearing every other word. You feel uncomfortable with this level of profanity. You would:

  _____ Cut short the visit by feigning illness (headaches work great for this purpose.)

  _____ Suffer silently and wait for the encounter to end.

  _____ Relate your discomfort to your friend and ask him or her to please moderate the use of these words.

Your solution

_____

_____

_____

Conclusion

There are many ways to react to life's insults. Our suggestion is to combine one part assertiveness, one part humor, and one part acceptance. That way if you can't change the situation once you have tried, you can either laugh about it or accept it. The key, of course, is first trying, then accepting.

The Directionality Exercise

This activity is _purposely_ designed to get you "on purpose" in life. We have an unusual point of view about purposes or life goals. Knowing your life goals means being able to answer the question "what it's all about" in general and "where I am going" in particular. Your first task is to determine whether you agree with our point of view.

We believe that if you went out in the street today and asked 100 people the question, "What are your purposes in life?" you would draw 97 blanks. You would discover that very few people have consciously thought through the values and myriad considerations involved in defining life goals. Yet an awareness of one's purposes is crucial for a wellness lifestyle.

Do you agree or not? Yes _____ No _____

Let's shift now for a close look at your purposes.

Please respond right off the top of your head to each of the following. Take no more than two minutes per question; let the first responses that come to mind flow right onto the page. Naturally, each question _deserves_ more time. However, the point here is to better identify, not develop, familiarity with purposes.

• What is your most important reason for living? Why is this number one? What are other major purposes in life for you?

_____

_____

_____

_____

_____

• Are these the same purposes in life your parents had? If not, what are the differences? How do you know there are differences?

_____

_____

_____

_____

_____

• Who has been most influential in stimulating you, in one way or another, to consider (i.e., to actively think about) life purposes?

_____

_____

_____

• What have you decided for yourself with respect to life purposes?

_____

_____

_____

• To what extent do your purposes reflect or bear on the kind of lifestyle you pursue? Explain.

_____

_____

_____

- Who serves on your "board of directors?" That is, who is running things? Rank the following forces with regard to the extent of influence which each, in its own way, exerts upon your attitudes and behaviors. Again, add whomever or whatever you wish to the list before doing the ranking.

  You _____

  Your children _____

  A quest or some kind of "manifest destiny" _____

  God _____

  Chance/fate/luck _____

  The government _____

  Your church/religion _____

  Parents _____

  Spouse _____

  Friends _____

  Job(s) _____

  _____

  _____

- Rank in order the following list of payoffs according to their importance to you. Before doing so, add a few items which we no doubt overlooked. (Interpret items any way you wish.)

  Sex _____

  Eating _____

  Athletic triumph _____

  Fame _____

  Acknowledgement/recognition _____

  Financial gain _____

  Spiritual advances _____

  Power _____

  _____

  _____

  _____

- What are you willing to give up or sacrifice for? On what occasions do you find yourself giving up pleasures? Why do you do this? (Make two columns: one for sacrifices, the other for brief explanations. As usual, allow only two minutes for responding to this question.)

Example:

Sacrifices/Postponed or Forfeited Desires	*Rationale for Doing So*
Banana Splits	They have too many calories; I will get fat if I eat them as often as I would like.
Taking a Caribbean cruise	Need to save the money for my children's education

_____

_____

_____

_____

- Is your self-esteem as high as you want it to be? If not, what will it take to raise it to a desired level?

  Perhaps the first step to wellness is self-love. No, not narcissism, but a genuine sense of caring for yourself. We label this caring self-esteem. A surprising large number of people, when asked the above question, have no notion at how to raise their self-esteem. Here are a few ideas:

  Make a list of your special qualities
  Note the self improvements that you have made over the last few years.
  Write down twenty things you like to do. Now check your list and determine when you last did them.
  Reflect on both the people and situations which have helped you raise your self-esteem in the past.

Improving self-esteem often involves reaching out, taking some risks, trying new ventures and learning new skills.

Without self-esteem the best of planning efforts may prove fruitless.

Interpretation

If you were comfortable in responding to these questions, if you found the activity relatively easy to complete, and if you feel reasonably satisfied with the uncensored replies to each query, then you are in a very good place! Your life has *directionality*. You are one of the three out of 100 whose actions and attitudes are in accord with chosen, aware purposes. If not, this activity should do you a lot of good. It will help you to examine and better come to terms with your own purposes.

Work on Yourself

Get determined to be well and happy. Don't expect someone else to do it for you. Since you have a great many self-images, play up those which support your move to wellness, and excuse the rest.

A truly free person should spend most of his/her time making wellness-oriented decisions, looking at trade-offs among positive alternatives. Do your best to maximize gains, rather than minimize losses when considering risks.

To escalate your planned shift toward wellness, consider some of the following strategies consistent with the goals you formulated in your personal wellness plan:

- Try new things, people, and places.
- Excuse yourself for not being perfect—it's not necessary.
- Expect worthwile change to take a while—otherwise the quest is too easy.
- Seek out adventure—such as romantic encounters.
- Don't be devastated by rejections, crises, awful weather, and unpleasant politicians—it's all part of the cycle. Better stuff is coming up.

Remember, for every problem, there is a solution that is simple, easy, and wrong! Work on finding your own answers—and do not expect that they will always be simple or easy. Let your thoughts be your guide to action—and use Planning for Wellness approaches to direct those thoughts toward wellness outcomes. In this way, you will guard against the problem expressed by John Dewey: "We are much more likely to act our way into a new way of thinking than we are to think our way into a new way of acting."

Conclusion

Reflecting on the many questions posed in Planning for Wellness should prove more valuable to you than settling on the answers. There is no scoring system.

The more you examine the internal workings of your own complexity, the better your prospects for meeting your true needs.

It's possible to learn a great deal from friends, as well as to be of service to them. By introducing these exercises as an after-dinner "game" or focus of discussion, you can (in a non-threatening, pressure-free way) create an opportunity for friends to examine the underpinnings of their own lifestyles. By serving others, you serve yourself. You alone are responsible for your choices, but wellness is most easily and enjoyably pursued in concert with others.

On this score, we have a final exercise for you: You have seen how planning for wellness at home, work, and play can open all kinds of possibilities for a richer, fuller and more satisfying life—in addition to the obvious health benefits.

How could you apply your individual commitment to personal excellence toward a larger advantage—to the benefit of the environment and to others whom you may never know or know of?

We have a technique that may apply. We call it "country and/or planetary goal setting." It has the effect of unleashing creativity and encouraging thoughts and ways that each of us could contribute to the larger scheme of things. This vision need not be totally down-to-earth. Not all of us are going to inspire statues in our image after our lifetimes, but why not think of grand terms once in a while?

Here is an example of what we have in mind. The following is the "country and/or planetary" goal of one Bernard Moitessier, as first reported in the French Newspaper Le/Figaro on April 23, 1980. Maybe it will inspire you to start thinking of a goal for the country and/or planet.

> I submit to you what I believe is a good idea—like something I have seen in a dream: to plant fruit trees along the streets of our towns, along all our roads and paths, in all our public parks, and even in our forests, for the species offer fine wood for construction and furniture, as well as edible fruit. For a fruit tree offers needed shade and greenery along with its fruits.
>
> But above all, these fruit trees, which would belong to everyone (including the birds and bees) without ownership by any particular person, would represent a symbol for the era of evolution which we must enter if we want to succeed in the building of the country and our planet.
>
> These fruit trees, while growing, could serve as a real and non-verbal participation in the creation of something much greater than our little selves, something generous and simple, which would help in uniting mankind in the spirit of an evolution of the wisdom of the heart.
>
> Mankind has built cathedrals. A country where the roads and walkways and streets were lined with fruit trees would, I believe, be even more beautiful than the most beautiful cathedral imaginable.

What might you like to do, someday, for the country and/or planet? Let your imagination play—and your heart go out. Don't be concerned about political feasibility, cost, and all that realistic stuff.

My Goal(s) _____

_____

_____

Parting Words

Wellness is a framework for the pursuit of a good and full life, close to the level of your potential, in concert with others similarly oriented. It is, however, just a framework, an attitude of mind and pattern of behavior; it is not an end in itself. "To travel hopefully is better than to arrive," as Parkinson observed.

Focus on what you can achieve, given where you are and want to go. Do not allow your earlier training to draw you toward complacence with limitations. Consider the case of W. Mitchell, Mayor of Crested Butte, who, though paralyzed from an air crash, maintains an ambitious schedule (and an impressive record of achievements on environmental issues). The Mayor's outlook on his disability exemplifies the truly healthy outlook on life.

> The way I look at it, before I was paralyzed, there were ten thousand things I could do; ten thousand things I was capable of doing. Now there are nine thousand. I can dwell on the one thousand, or concentrate on the nine thousand I have left. And, of course the joke is that none of us in our lifetime is going to do more than two or three thousand of these things in any event.*

Concentrate on the thousands of ways that are available to you for bringing about wellness at home, work, and play.

We have no further advice save this parting announcement:

> The elevator to wellness is out of order!
> Take the stairs.
> Breathe deeply after climbing each level.
> Enjoy the view.

Be well.

---

*Quoted in *Options: Spinal Cord Injuries and the Future,* by Barry Corbet. Published by National Spinal Cord Injury Foundation, 369 Elliot Street, Newton Upper Falls, Maine, 02164, p. 32, 1980.

Bibliography

Self-Responsibility

- Ardell, Donald B. *High Level Wellness: An Alternative to Doctors, Drugs and Disease.* Emmaus, PA: Rodale Press, 1977, and New York: Bantam, 1979.
- Ardell, Donald B. *14 Days to a Wellness Lifestyle.* Mill Valley: Whatever Press, 1982.
- Clark, Carolyn Chambers. *Enhancing Wellness: A Guide for Self-Care.* New York: Springer Publishing Co., 1981.
- Farquhar, John W. *The American Way of Life Need Not Be Hazardous to Your Health.* New York: Norton, 1978.
- Ferguson, Tom. *Medical Self Care: Access to Self-Help Tools.* New York: Simon and Schuster, 1980.
- Ryan, Regina Sara and Travis, John W. *The Wellness Workbook.* Berkeley, CA: Ten Speed Press, 1981.
- Tager, Mark and Jennings, Charles. *Whole-Person Health Care.* Portland, OR: Victoria House, 1978.
- Vickery, Donald M. *Lifeplan for Your Health.* Reading, Pa: Addison-Wesley, 1978.

Nutritional Awareness

- Ballentine, Rudolph. *Diet and Nutrition: A Holistic Approach.* Honesdale, PA: Himalayan Institute, 1978.
- *Dietary Goals for the United States.* Senate Select Committee on Nutrition and Human Needs. Washington, D.C.: U.S. Government Printing Office, 1977.
- Gerras, Charles, et al. *The Complete Book of Vitamins.* Emmaus, PA: Rodale Press, 1977.
- Hewitt, J. *The New York Times Natural Foods Cookbook.* New York: Avon, 1972.
- Nutrition Search, Inc. *Nutrition Almanac* (2nd ed.). New York: McGraw-Hill, 1979.
- Osman, Jack D. *Thin From Within: Vegetarian Edition.* Washington, D.C.: Review and Herald Publishing Association, 1981.
- Pritikin, Nathan, et al. *The Pritikin Program for Diet and Exercise.* New York: Grossett & Dunlap, 1979.
- Kasen, R. *That First Bite: Journal of a Compulsive Overeater.* New York: Pomerica, 1979.
- Williams, Roger. *The Wonderful World Within You: Your Inner Nutritional Environment.* New York: Bantam, 1977.

Stress Awareness and Management

- Bloomfield, Harold H. and Kory, Robert B. *The Holistic Way to Health and Happiness.* New York: Simon and Schuster, 1978.
- Davis, M. *The Relaxation and Stress Reduction Workbook.* San Francisco: New Harbinger Publishers, 1980.
- Dychtwald, Ken. *Body Mind.* New York: Jove, 1978.
- Hastings, Arthur C., et. al. *Health for the Whole Person: The Complete Guide to Holistic Medicine.* Boulder: Westview Press, 1980.
- Gawain, Shakti. *Creative Visualizations.* Mill Valley, CA: Whatever Publishing, 1981.
- Pelletier, Kenneth R. *Mind as Healer, Mind as Slayer: A Holistic Approach to Preventing Stress Disorders.* New York, Delta, 1977.
- Schafer, Walt. *Stress, Distress & Growth.* Davis, CA: International Dialogue Press, 1978.
- Tubesing, Donald A. *Kicking Your Stress Habits.* Duluth, MN, Whole Person Associates, 1981.

Physical Fitness

- Anderson, Bob. *Stretching.* Fullerton, California, 1975.
- Bailey, Covert. *Fit or Fat.* Boston: Houghton-Mifflin, 1978.
- Fixx, Jim. *Jim Fixx's Second Book of Running.* New York: Random House, 1980.
- Galloway, Tim and Kriegal, Bob. *Inner Skiing.* New York: Bantam, 1979.
- Kuntzleman, Charles. *Activetics.* New York: Wydan, 1978.

Environmental Sensitivity

- Allen, Robert F. *Lifegain.* New York: Appleton-Century Crofts, 1981.
- Dyer, Wayne W. *Your Erroneous Zones.* New York: Avon, 1976.
- Emery, Stewart. *Actualizations: You Don't Have to Rehearse To Be Yourself.* New York: Dolphin Books, 1978.
- Maslow, Abraham. *Toward a Psychology of Being.* New York: Van Nostrand, 1968.
- Segal, Jeanne. *Feeling Great: Enhancing Your Health and Well Being.* Santa Cruz: Orenda/Unity Press, 1981.
- Sher, Barbara. *Wishcraft: How To Get What You Really Want,* New York: Viking, 1979.
- Vickery, Donald M. *Life Plan For Your Health.* Reading, M.A.: Addison-Wesley, 1978.
- Yankelovich, Daniel. *New Rules: Searching for Self-Fulfillment in a World Turned Upside Down.* New York: Random House, 1981.

Goal and Activity Sheet

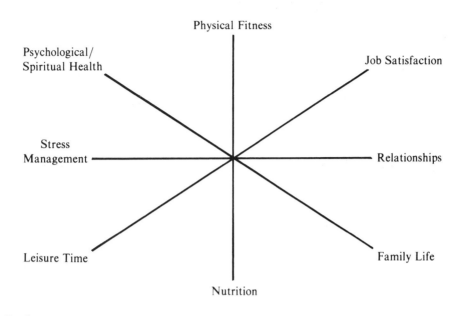

Physical Fitness

Psychological/
Spiritual Health

Job Satisfaction

Stress
Management

Relationships

Leisure Time

Family Life

Nutrition

I. Goal: _____

_____

Activities: _____

_____

II. Goal: _____

_____

Activities: _____

_____

III. Goal: _____

_____

Activities: _____

_____

IV. Goal: _____

_____

Activities: _____

_____

Contract

I, _____ do hereby commit myself to the following goals and activities for _____ weeks. This agreement with myself should be in effect from _____ until _____ .

- The goals I set for myself are:

_____

_____

_____

_____

- To pursue these goals, I will perform the following activities on a regular basis. Specifically, the time set aside for each goal is as follows: (Note both the goal-related activity and when it will be performed.)

_____

_____

_____

_____

- Friends who will assist me in these pursuits are:

_____

_____

- I realize I may sabotage my plan by:

_____

_____

- So I will avoid this by:

_____

_____

- The payoffs which I will realize by fulfilling my goals are:

_____

_____

_____

Signed _____ Date _____

Witness _____

Goal and Activity Sheet

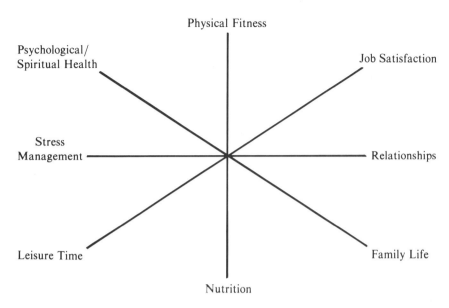

I. Goal: _____

_____

Activities: _____

_____

II. Goal: _____

_____

Activities: _____

_____

III. Goal: _____

_____

Activities: _____

_____

IV. Goal: _____

_____

Activities: _____

_____

Contract

I, _____ do hereby commit myself to the following goals and activities for _____ weeks. This agreement with myself should be in effect from _____ until _____ .

- The goals I set for myself are:

  _____

  _____

  _____

  _____

- To pursue these goals, I will perform the following activities on a regular basis. Specifically, the time set aside for each goal is as follows: (Note both the goal-related activity and when it will be performed.)

  _____

  _____

  _____

  _____

- Friends who will assist me in these pursuits are:

  _____

  _____

- I realize I may sabotage my plan by:

  _____

  _____

- So I will avoid this by:

  _____

  _____

- The payoffs which I will realize by fulfilling my goals are:

  _____

  _____

  _____

Signed _____ Date _____

Witness _____

Graphs

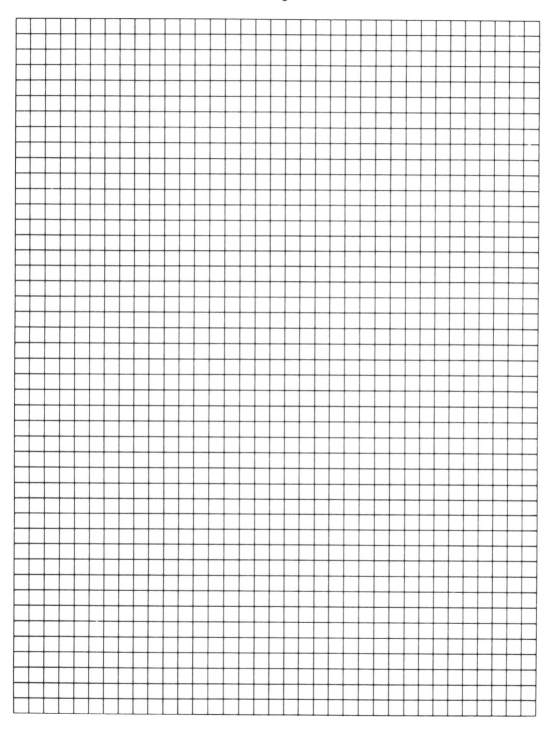

Graphs

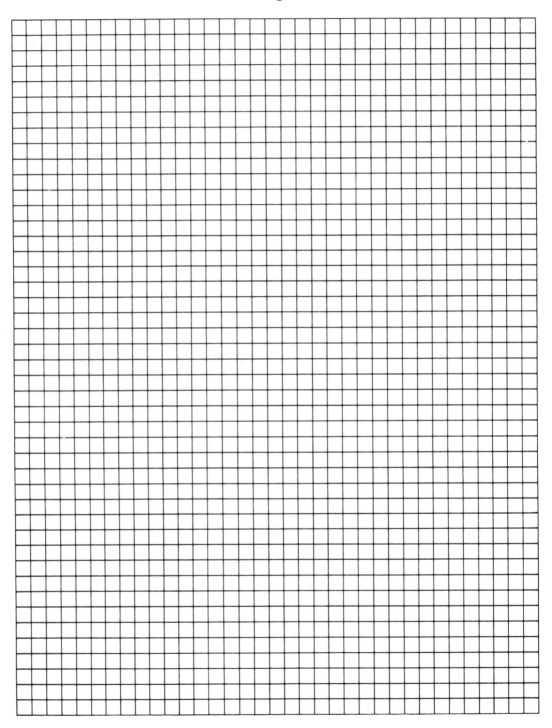

Graphs

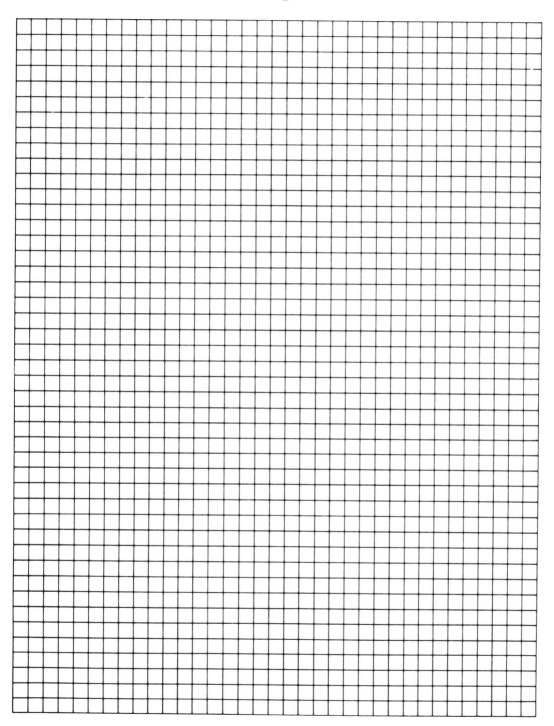

Graphs

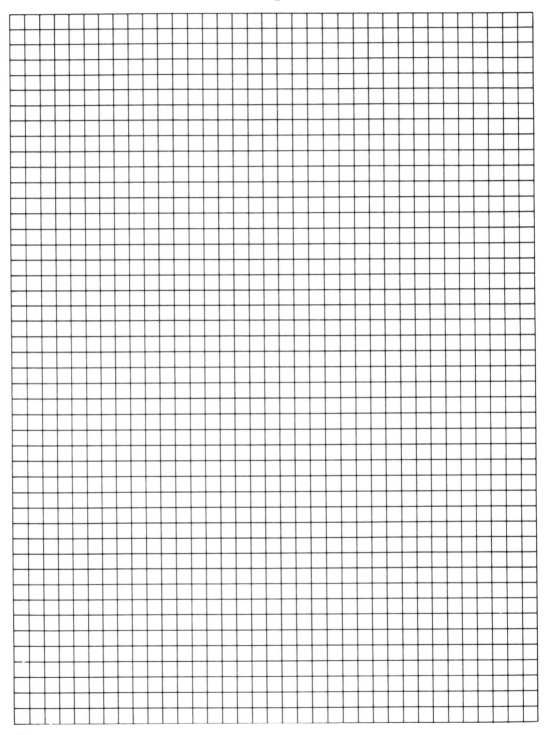

Graphs

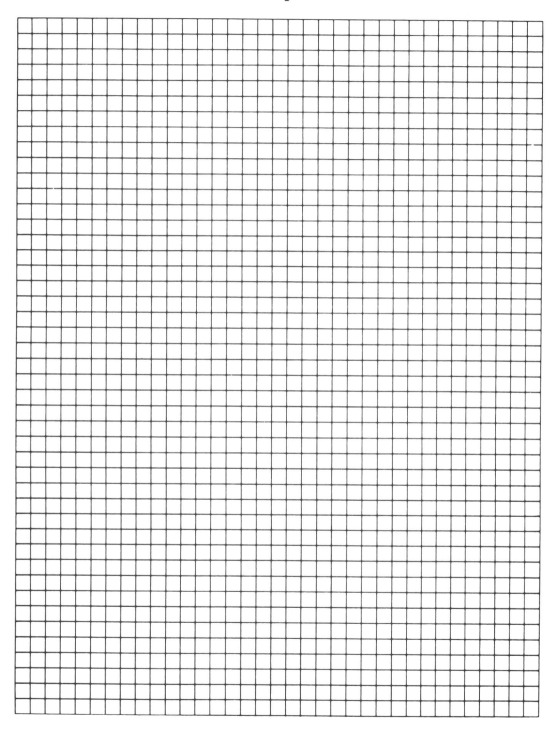

Graphs

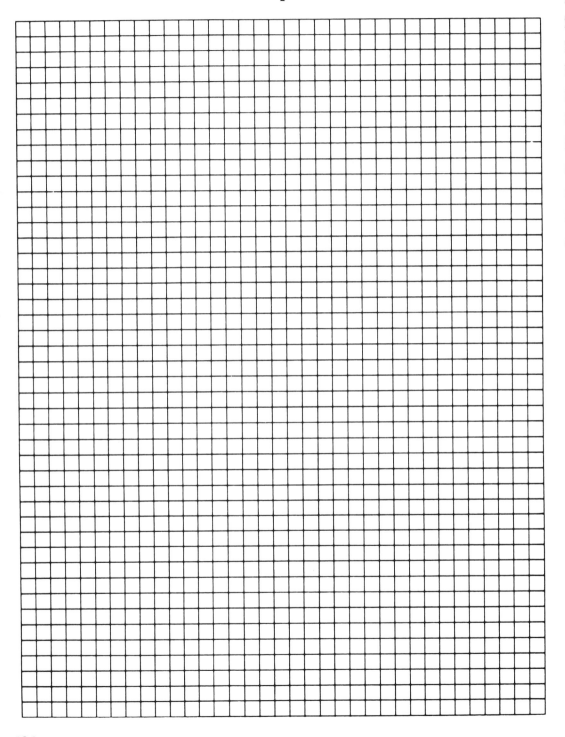

Available Supportive Film Material

"A Personal Plan for Wellness" is designed to accompany the acclaimed guidebook *Planning For Wellness*. It conveys, through a fanciful situation comedy, the nature and rewards of a wellness lifestyle in order to motivate the viewer to give the personal plan approach a try.

It should be especially effective with young people, participants in corporate health promotion programs, and for anyone interested in learning how to improve his or her level of physical and psychological well-being.

This 25 minute film is available in video tape and 16 mm. For additional information please write:

Marketing Dept.
Kendall/Hunt Publishing Co.
2460 Kerper Blvd.
Dubuque, Iowa 52001